IRRADIATION
of Mice and Men

IRRADIATION

of Mice and Men

John F. Loutit

THE UNIVERSITY OF CHICAGO PRESS

Library of Congress Catalog Card Number: 62-12635

THE UNIVERSITY OF CHICAGO PRESS, CHICAGO & LONDON
The University of Toronto Press, Toronto 5, Canada

PREFACE

Who decides what is a reasonable dose of radiation for you, John Citizen, to receive from radioactive material in your backyard, or for you, Archie Artisan, from the industrial X-ray machine which is the tool of your trade? The answer is the International Commission on Radiological Protection.

This is perhaps a unique organization. In the nineteen-twenties the radiologists in many countries, and especially Great Britain, realized that all was not well with their conditions of work. Observation and experiment had shown that X-rays could be a cause not only of acute local damage to the patient but of serious disease in the radiologist chronically exposed. Local committees examined the hazards and how to minimize them. In 1928 representatives of these national bodies got together at the International Congress of Radiology to form the International Commission with members selected, not like the United National Assembly from every country represented, but for their personal expertise irrespective of nationality and, incredible as it may seem now, responsible for their own expenses.

This International Commission meeting every three years at successive congresses and its national counterparts rapidly put in order the houses where medical radiology was carried out.

From 1942, when the first self-sustaining reaction of nuclear fission was effected in Chicago, radiation hazards became a problem, not of the small department in the basement of the hospital or of the university laboratory, but of the vast enterprise. Due to the forethought of the International Commission and its national counterparts, the principles and codes of practice could be expanded and applied immediately. Indeed, the industrial history of nuclear energy in the last 20 years has been singularly good in terms of freedom from accidents and occupationally induced illness despite the tremendous potential hazards.

When international congresses could meet again after World War II, the International Commission took up and extended its former role to take account of the extensive new problems. These involve not only external irradiation with a variety of nuclear particles as well as electromagnetic radiations but internal irradiation from man-made radioactive nucleides. In this task it has recently received financial support from a number of organizations including the Ford Foundation. The principle of membership remains, as before, the election of the expert for his personal qualifications.

At the national level there is naturally variation from country to country. In Great Britain the government relies for advice and guidance in such matters on the Medical Research Council who in turn are advised by a Committee on Protection against Ionizing Radiations. The members of this Committee are likewise selected for their personal knowledge and listed in the Medical Research Council's Annual Report.

This practice of the British government has recently received some criticism in the *New Scientist* from Geminus* who writes:

> The point I wish to make is that the Government habitually expects too much of the MRC, and that the Council shoulders too much of the public responsibility when it sets out to promulgate "maximum permissible doses" of radiation of various kinds.
>
> For by now there is no doubt that many of the biological effects of radiation can be caused by quite small doses. In principle, then, the only way in which a "permissible level" of radiation dose can be chosen is by balancing the advantages to society of some particular use of radiation against its possible biological disadvantages. The difficulty is, of course, that of balancing such considerations against each other. As the mathematicians say, they are really incommensurable. It would, for instance, take a battalion of Solomons working a 48-hour week for ten years on end to tell exactly how the balance should be struck between the advantages of building nuclear power stations and the risks that radiation from these installations will necessarily entail.
>
> Unfortunately the fact that these questions are difficult does not excuse the way in which the politicians have run away from them. Indeed, there is some cause for saying that the art of politics lies precisely in the making

New Scientist, Dec. 7, 1961.

of compromises between incommensurable considerations. Yet nobody in public life seems squarely to have faced the question of how great a biological risk should be entailed for the sake of this or that use of radiation.

In these circumstances it is courageous of the MRC to have added this almost ethical task to its duty of providing a technical assessment of the risks of radiation in its various uses. Moreover, it has done its extra chore cautiously, with the scales well weighted in favour of people. But, I think, the time has long passed when responsibility should be passed back to the place where it belongs.

Similar questions could arise about the rectitude of relying on the International Commission on Radiological Protection for decisions which can be claimed as political. I have the unmitigated effrontery to hold that this is not an ordinary political problem involving the balance of vested interests. In principle the same can be said about most problems involving health, but the known chemical and biological noxa can be better localized and controlled. The practical problems connected with operations in nuclear energy on a large scale concern the release of radioactive materials, many of them with long half-lives of their radioactivity. There is no way of inactivating radioactivity or shortening its active period. There is no practical method of preventing its spread in the atmosphere or oceans once it has escaped from containment. Thus standards of radioactive contamination and hygiene are of more than parochial or national interest.

To me, therefore, the principle of radiation-protection is something to be judged wherever practicable by absolute rather than relative standards. Consequently there is an overwhelming case for these principles to be considered by a panel of experts unbiased by national, financial, or other "political" factors.

Whatever the future, however, there is a profound need for a general understanding among the politically conscious of what is known and unknown of the biological effects of radiation and their implications. The Rockefeller Foundation has provided financial support to the Section of Nuclear Medicine in the Department of Pharmacology of the University of Chicago for such constructive criticism and dissemination of information. It was with this term of reference that I was privileged to give the subsequent lectures at the University in October, 1961.

I wish to thank Drs. Harvey M. Patt of the Argonne National Laboratory, Hardin B. Jones of the Donner Laboratory, the University of California, and Franklin C. McLean of the University of Chicago, who served as moderators at the lectures, for their stimulating discussions. I am indebted to my colleague, Dr. C. E. Ford, for Figs. 1–11 and I gratefully acknowledge that the motivating force behind me in the preparation and delivery of these lectures was Dr. John H. Rust of the University of Chicago.

CONTENTS

ILLUSTRATIONS

CHAPTER ONE

RADIATION
AND THE FACTS OF LIFE

Apologia

The sponsors of these lectures have invited me to discuss the problems of the biological hazards of nuclear energy in my capacity as a radiobiologist. This title suggests that I am a specialist; and indeed I discover that many of the young men I meet in laboratories, when I inquire of their special interest and expertise, say radiobiology. In contrast, to me and my closest associates radiobiology is the inverse of a specialty. It implies to us as a prerequisite a knowledge of the whole of biology and as a consequence an understanding of the alteration of function following exposure to radiation. However, the "good old days" of, say, two hundred years ago, when an educated man could be elected to the Royal Society and be expected to be expert in all fields of science, have long since departed. In this century we must rely on the committee of wise men; our descendants will probably place more reliance on electronic brains.

Thus I recognize that in the following dissertation I may commit some nonsense, for the scientist is no more immune from this fault than the consultant in other walks of life.

The Physical Nature of the Hazard

IONIZING RADIATIONS

In the last half-dozen years there has been a widespread public apprehension of the hazards connected with the increasing use of ionizing radiation. As the least of my specialties is nuclear physics, I shall not enlarge on the nice distinction between ionizing and non-ionizing radiations. However, I can propound that ionizing radiations are of many kinds. Some consist of particles, electrically charged like α- and β-rays or uncharged like neutrons; some consist of electromagnetic rays, for example X and γ, forming an extension of the spectrum of such radiations, which include heat and light, to rays of very short wave length. The common feature of both the particulate and electromagnetic radiations in question is their capacity to cause the ejection of atomic particles from the atoms or molecules in which some or all of their energy is absorbed.

ROLE OF RADIATIONS IN NATURE

A supply of energy is necessary for the growth and maintenance of life in all biological cells, but on this planet the source of energy is derived from chemical processes (hence biochemistry), though the biological function may be manifested as an output of physical energy (hence biophysics). In the form of heat physical energy may supplement the chemical sources of energy by speeding up the chemical reactions or, in the case of man, by counteracting heat loss from the body: in the form of light it initiates the most important biological process on earth—photosynthesis; but fundamentally the biological cell ticks from chemical energy. While heat and light are essential in the environment of Earth's biota, there is as yet no conclusive evidence that ionizing radiations have any similar role. Notwithstanding this, no life has existed without ionizing radiation, since the Earth is mildly radioactive from the presence of a few very long-lived, naturally radioactive elements and isotopes of stable elements and since ionizing radiation in the form of cosmic radiation reaches the Earth's surface from outer space. We cannot exclude in the present state of knowledge that traces, as it were, of ionizing radiation subserve some useful, or even necessary, function, just as traces of some chemical elements are necessary as micronutrients. The essential trace-elements are usually constituents of enzymes, those biological catalysts which facilitate chemical reactions. A deficiency of trace-elements results in impairment of biological activity, even death; an excess may easily produce equally serious intoxication; and the optima lie in a band of variable dimensions between the two extremes. For ionizing radiations all our information is concerned with the so-called radiotoxic effects.

THE BIOLOGICAL TARGETS

The living things of the Earth range from unicellular organisms up to highly complex vertebrates, with mammals and, we think, man at the top of the evolutionary tree. In the unicellular organism all the functions necessary for maintenance and reproduction are represented in the cell. To some this represents a relatively simple system, and its natural physiological functions and altered reactions after irradiation or other insult are the object of their study. To others the specialization of groups of cells into tissues in multi-cellular organisms, which has occurred in evolutionary development, represents a simplification and allows more defined investigation of specific processes, complicated though it may be by the need to consider the interdependence of the different constituent tissues which make up the entire organism. The multiplicity of views is acceptable and desirable. As a consequence, if some reaction is found to be common to the single cell and to a tissue, and especially if it is common to different tissues, that reaction can be taken as a biological law. The difficulty lies in the interpretation of reactions which are limited to certain systems or conditions.

In general, Nature has been prodigal with her gifts. The individual cell, be it the self-dependent unicellular organism or the unit of a tissue, has been endowed with an abundance of machinery as capital. In the same way tissues are usually provided with an excess of cells above the minimal or normal requirements and with a wide margin of reproductive potential. There are exceptions, however, to these generalizations.

In the case of the cell the only well-known example of paucity of essential substance concerns the genes, the units of inheritable material which control specific biochemical processes. The diploid cells of most higher organisms have only two homologous genes. For sexually reproducing organisms, one gene of the pair is derived from each parent. Simple organisms may be haploid and have only one gene of each variety. Any loss of a gene or molecular change, the so-called mutation, is thus likely to have profound results as far as that particular cell is concerned, certainly if it is haploid, possibly if it is diploid, but less likely if it is polyploid.

When the tissue is considered, the consequences of loss or change in an individual cell depend upon its natural life span. If the tissue is one which has naturally a high rate of turnover of cells, such as the skin or blood-forming bone marrow, the effect is trivial. The normal replicative machinery can expand its output to cover all but exceptionally large losses. This could be by a shortening of the turnover-time, that is a speeding-up of the rate of division, or by an expansion of work space. For instance, the active bone marrow in the normal adult occupies but half the total available space; under the appropriate stress it can expand into the whole.

On the other hand certain tissues, like the liver of the normal adult, have little or no natural turnover of cells, but, given accidental destruction of part of the liver, the remainder is activated to effect the replacement. So once again a limited loss of cells is of minor consequence only.

There remain, however, some specialized cells which are irreplaceable in the adult mammal. Nerve cells and oöcytes, partially mature egg cells of the female, are in this category. Loss of these cells *is* important. Most female mammals have been provided with more oöcytes than would be good for them to convert into ova for fertilization and production of offspring, and many are probably lost spontaneously; but given an accidental loss the reserve can be called upon. This reserve, it is important to remember, is limited. In contrast, nerve cells, according to current dogma,

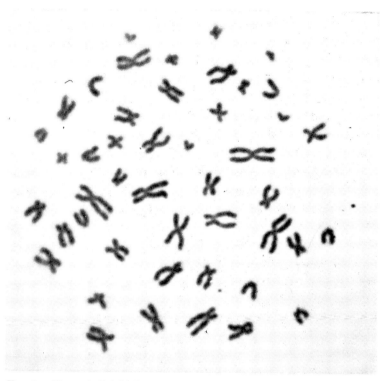

FIG. 1.—Normal diploid ($2n = 46$) set of chromosomes in a cell from the bone marrow of a human female. $\times$ 3700.

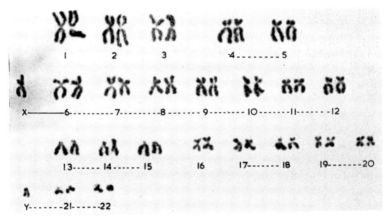

Fig. 2.—Karyotype of a normal human male.

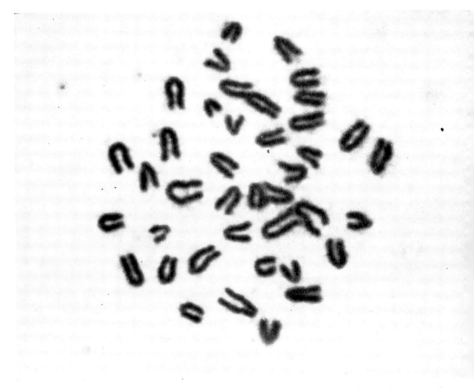

Fig. 3.—Chromosomes ($2n = 40$) of a cell from the spleen of a normal mouse. $\times 2700$.

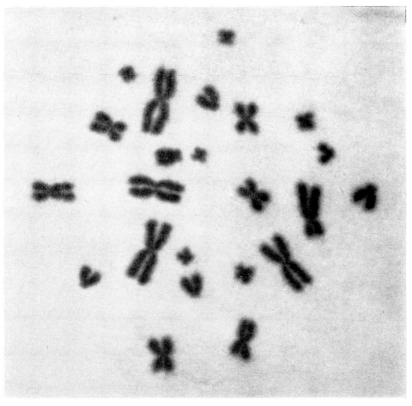

FIG. 4.—Normal diploid (2n = 22) set of chromosomes in a cell from the
spleen of a Chinese hamster. × 2700

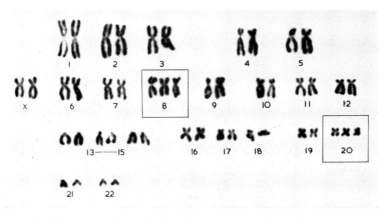

FIG. 5.—Karyotype of a cell with 48 chromosomes from the bone marrow
of a human subject with blast-cell (acute) leukemia.

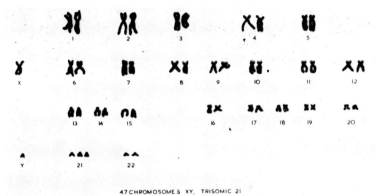

47 CHROMOSOMES XY, TRISOMIC 21

Fig. 6.—Karyotype of a male mongoloid imbecile.

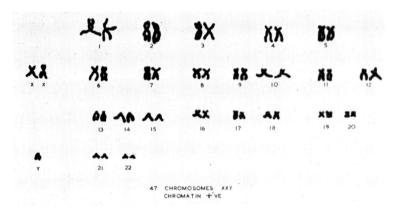

47 CHROMOSOMES XXY
CHROMATIN +'VE

Fig. 7.—Karyotype of a male with Klinefelter's syndrome (chromatin—positive).

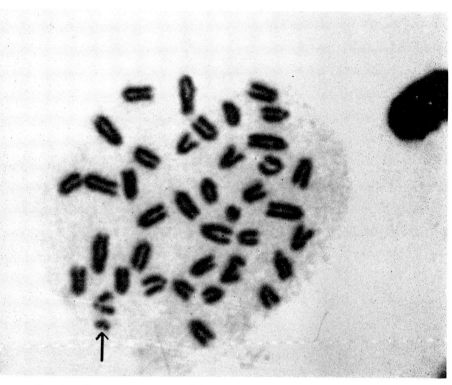

Fig. 8.—Chromosomes in a cell from the thymus of a mouse heterozygous for the T6 translocation. The arrow points to the small marker chromosome. × 2700.

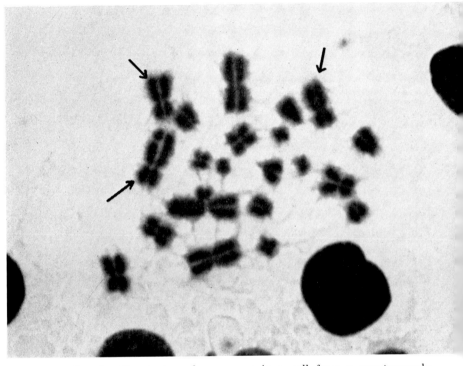

Fig. 9.—Twenty-two chromosomes in a cell from a spontaneously arising primary reticulosarcoma in a Chinese hamster. Three marker chromosomes are indicated by arrows. × 2700.

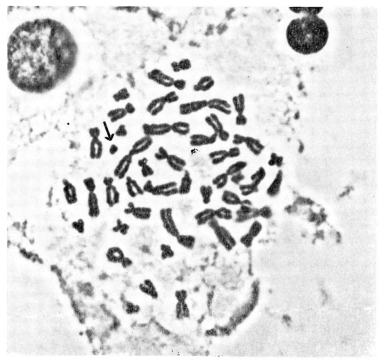

FIG. 10.—Chromosomes (46) in a cultured white blood cell from a human subject. The arrow points to the small "Philadelphia" chromosome. × 3200.

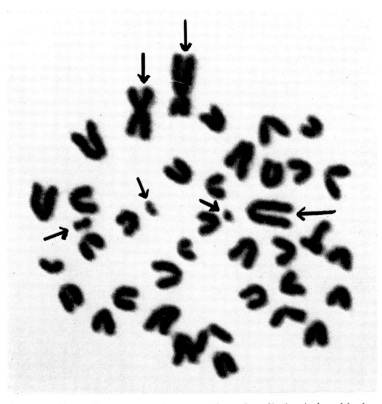

Fig. 11.—Forty chromosomes in a transplanted, radiation-induced leukemic cell. There are 6 marker chromosomes (arrows). × 3500.

are all performing an essential service, and any loss is followed by a corresponding loss of function. Depending on the specialized site and performance of the nerve cells, this may entail loss of perceptive sense, loss of motor power, loss of co-ordination, or loss of those higher central functions of thought and reasoning which raise man above other mammals and mammals above the "bird brains." It is true that one may compensate for limited loss of nerve cells by use of alternative pathways. The nervous system is one for communication and can be compared with a network of roads. The destruction of several lengths of road does not necessarily lead to significant loss of communication, but roads can be repaired while nerve cells cannot. The importance of the nervous system is therefore obvious. It may be that in Britain and the U.S.A. we have underrated potential effects of ionizing radiation and other damaging agents on the nervous system and consequently on the total body economy. Certainly structural damage observable with the naked eye or the conventional light microscope is not visible in the majority of instances. Our physiological and medical colleagues in the U.S.S.R. on the other hand, since the days of Pavlov, have tended to incriminate the nervous system as the seat of many disorders, even when structural changes are minimal and arguable, on the grounds of functional disturbance manifested by electrophysiological disturbances and aberrations of behavior. The whole subject is an area where lack of agreement between scientists is understandable. Our anatomical approach has been through the relatively crude methods hitherto available and may have resulted in the scoring of many false negatives. By contrast, the electrophysiological and behavioristic approach is open to many false positives.

Nature of Radiotoxic Effect

For half a century interest has been focused on the capacity of ionizing radiation to inhibit or prevent cell division. When radiobiology, a generation ago, was stimulated almost solely by the efforts of the radiotherapist to kill cancers, which are composed of rapidly growing but more or less atypical primitive cells, this was natural, for if cell division could be stopped the cancer cells would be frustrated. They would either have to die a natural death or mature as do primitive cells of a normal lineage.

This must not be taken to imply that our fathers were unaware of other toxic actions of these radiations. They merely judged that the greatest rewards for their efforts would be in the study of radiation-effects in cell division. The majority verdict today does not seem very different.

As long ago as 1906 the effects of a substantial dose of X-rays delivered to a whole animal were recognized as being most obviously on those tissues which were actively dividing. The law of Bergonié and Tribondeau states:

. . . X-rays are more effective on cells which have greater reproductive activity; the effectiveness is greater on those cells which have a longer dividing future ahead, on those cells the morphology and the function of which are least fixed. From this law it is easy to understand that roentgen radiation destroys tumors without destroying healthy tissues [1].

CELL DEATH

The minority today are impressed with the exception rather than the rule. Amongst the extremely radiosensitive cells of the mammal are lymphocytes. These make up the characteristic cell population of lymphoid tissue, which forms discrete nodes (lymph glands) and aggregates in various tissues, notably spleen and intestinal mucosa. The thymus gland, which is still largely a mystery, is also part of the system. Lymphocytes are classified as large, medium, and small, and the small are generally agreed to be the mature form which are the end of the developmental chain and are non-dividing. Nevertheless they are as radiosensitive as any cell in the body. The radiotoxic effect cannot be mediated by disruption of their reproductive mechanism. It is apparently the nucleus which is affected; within an hour or so of irradiation loss of the normal nuclear pattern is seen on microscopic examination and complete dissolution soon follows.

This direct and early radiotoxic effect is not peculiar to lymphocytes. When looked for, it can be seen in irradiated cancer cells, spermatogonia in the testis, erythroblasts in the bone marrow, oöcytes, and retinal cells in the eye of newborn mice. A case has been made by my colleagues in Oxford (Ord and Stocken [2]) that this is due to a "biochemical lesion" with disruption of the supply of chemical energy for nuclear metabolism. Effects of this sort can be scored in lymphoid cells with a dose as low as 5 r (Trowell [3]) or spermatogonia (Oakberg [4]).

CELL DIVISION

The classical effect of radiation is on the cell which is due to divide. Cell division by the process of mitosis in the somatic cells insures the perpetuation of the cell species by a doubling of the cellular, especially nuclear, material and the exact sharing of the products to the two daughter cells produced. Cell division in germ cells has to be different (meiosis) at a certain stage in order to effect a reduction to half of the nuclear material. Thus when fertilization of the female egg moiety occurs by the male half, the spermatozoon, the resulting zygote has the normal complement. Naturally these exquisitely delicate operations are susceptible to disturbance. There is abundant evidence now that "spontaneous" errors occur with a low but measurable frequency. What radiation and certain toxic chemicals do is to increase the chance of error.

It is not necessary here to describe what is known about mitotic and meiotic division and what is still obscure. A good account in simple language has been given by Alexander (5). Let it suffice to say that the structural unit of nuclear material is the chromosome. This is not visible as such in the nucleus for most of the cell's life cycle but manifests itself during the process of division, especially well at the midtime or metaphase. Then it can be seen that different species have a characteristic number of chromosomes, 46 for man (Figs. 1 and 2), 40 for the mouse (Fig. 3), and 42 for the rhesus monkey. Most eutherian mammals have these large numbers, though the Chinese hamster makes do with 22 (Fig. 4) and marsupials get by with a similar number or less. Many plants have still fewer numbers in a cell which is much larger than the mammal's. Thus chromosome cytology was largely the botanist's province till a few years ago. Now with recent improvements in technique, in which a notable role has been played by my colleague, Charles Ford, who started life as a botanist, mammalian cells can be studied with but little less accuracy.

Given the improved technique, it can now be seen that a substantial number of clinical syndromes are associated with visible abnormalities of the chromosomes. For the last year practically every issue of the medical weekly journal *Lancet* has contained reports of these which can broadly be divided into two categories. The first includes some cancers and like malignant conditions (Fig. 5). Indeed it had long been known from conventional histology that this could be so, but the modern techniques have permitted much greater definition. The second and more exciting is a miscellany of defects of development of the nervous system and of the sex glands often with defects in other systems (Fig. 6), and, in the case of sex glands, with secondary side effects (Fig. 7). In some subjects all the cells examined are alike, suggesting that the effect stemmed from the zygote and involved one or other of the parental halves; in other subjects, the so-called mosaics, two kinds of cells are scored, indicating a fault in one of the very early divisions of the developing embryo. Most of these abnormalities of development are attributed to non-disjunction; that is, in one division, when the two sets of chromosomes separate to their respective poles, one chromosome gets into the wrong lobby, so that in meiosis a germ cell with 24 or 22 chromosomes instead of 23 results.

The chromosomes are the carriers of the genes. At one time the genes were envisaged as something like large molecular beads arranged on the string of the chromosomes in a definite order. The ordering and orderliness of genes are capable of experimental verification in animals which are well categorized genetically, such as drosophila and mice; but the beads-on-a-string hypothesis is perhaps rather naïve. Now, in an attempt to explain matters in biochemical terms, genes are presumed to be codings within desoxyribonucleic acid molecules.

Presumably the gene-molecular complex, whatever it be, can be subject to purely local effects resulting in gene-mutation, which in turn results in a change of the function determined by that gene. A disturbance of greater magnitude can have more extensive effects with rupture of the chromosome substance. These breaks are well established. They may involve the whole chromosome or, when it has undergone duplication prior to division, only one of its two subunits. Union is the common sequel, just as it is with fractured bones, but, like untreated fractures of bones, the union may not be optimal; bits may get left out (deletions), bits may get back to front (inversions), and wrong bits may get included (translocations) (Fig. 8). It must be inevitable then with such patent structural lesions that the contained genes must be damaged too. It comes as no surprise, therefore, that the reconstructed unit is less competent than the original.

Nevertheless some of these reconstructed chromosomes function very adequately, and the cell's function is apparently as good as usual. The real test comes when the cell has to divide. If one or more of the essential parts of the replicative mechanism have been damaged or lost, the cell may not be able to complete the operation, and the products are removed and dissolved. This occurs at the first division when the damage has been calamitous or, following less serious damage, at the second or third division. Only the least serious are permanently viable.

This appears to be the state of the chromosomes of many tumors. With non-disjunction the chromosomes are too many or too few, but individually they are indistinguishable by present techniques from the standard. In malignant cells, on the other hand, chromosomes of identifiably abnormal form may be present (Fig. 9). Since with the light microscope we can see but little of the intimate detail of chromosomes, we could speculate that all malignant cells had similar but less obvious structural faults. This might lead to the further deduction that the malignant cell was a mutant form of the normal.

"Somatic mutation" has been invoked many times in the past, and still is today, as the cause of cancer; and probably structural change in the chromosome with associated involvement of genes is a more realistic concept than pure gene-mutation. Austin Brues (6) has summarized the arguments against this facile hypothesis. I would merely add the note of logic: even if all malignant cells exhibit chromosomal damage (which has not yet been shown), this could equally well be a result rather than a cause of the malignant state, and there is much to be said for this view. First of all, the lesions are very variable between malignancies of the same apparent type—the exception to this is the recently noted "Philadelphia chromosome" (7) of chronic myeloid leukemia (Fig. 10). Second, in experimental animals it is possible to follow changes in the malignant cells with time in the original host and serially in genetically identical animals of the same strain (Fig. 11); the cell population varies from time to time and different variants predominate at different times, apparently a selection of the fittest.

Surely, too, it is a mistake to talk of the cause of cancer, for cancers are as variable in character—namely site, form, growth, and age of onset—as individuals or as species. What they have in common is a lack of response to the normal discipline of the body.

I have ranged rather far over some of the normal facts of life as a necessary background to the effects of radiation. Cell division is an essential process to normal development and maintenance of an organism. It is a delicate operation with a small but definite chance of fault or failure each time. What radiation does is to magnify the incidence of fault. Does it produce a specific fault which is recognizable infallibly as caused by radiation? The answer is as far as we know—no.

Non-disjunction as a natural phenomenon is now a subject of the very greatest moment. Radiation has long been known to "cause" non-disjunction, but the range of qualitative effects and the quantitative relationships have not been explored to any extent yet. Undoubtedly the stimulus has now been given.

Breakage of chromosomes by radiation has been the subject of extensive study for a generation or more. A single localized event such as an ionization is not sufficient to cause breakage, but a series of events may well be. Thus the passage of a densely ionizing particle will do it. Protons and α-particles ejected from matter by neutrons have the necessary densely ionizing property and so have slow electrons, those of intrinsically low energy or fast electrons at the end of their tracks, whereas the fast electrons elsewhere on their rather errant route ionize but sparsely. To produce this sort of damage, the tracks of fast electrons have to summate one with another or several at the same time, that is, the intensity of radiation or dose-rate has to be high and the so-called two-hit effect must occur in contrast to the one-hit effect of the densely ionizing radiations, where effect is proportional to dose irrespective of time.

It is tremendously important to recognize the time factor. Often one hears of "recovery" from the effects of X- and γ-rays, which depend for their action on the liberation of fast electrons in the tissues in which they are absorbed, and of no "recovery" from the effects of neutrons that liberate protons. Thus 1,000 r of X-rays given in a single dose in 10 minutes (100 r/min) will kill a mouse within 10 days by destroying virtually all its blood-forming cells; 1,000 r given at uniform low dose-rate over 28 days (0.025 r/min) will have little immediate effect. Recuperative powers have been invoked because the tissue has survived 1,000 r. The dose is the same in the two instances, it is true, but the dose-rates differ by 4,000-fold. Not only is the damage entirely different due to this time factor with X-rays, but the cell population is entirely different too. Any cells killed or damaged due to chance can have been replaced with offspring of other cells which also by chance have escaped damage altogether or have received non-lethal injury.

In a similar way, 1,000 r may be given at high intensity (100 r/min) but in fractions spread out in time, perhaps over 28 days in 4 fractions of 250 r or in daily fractions of 36 r. Again the mouse will survive the immediate effects. In these instances the dose-rate is the same as when the 1,000 r was given in 10 minutes, but the over-all time is varied, and the cell populations irradiated are not the same. True recovery may occur but it is difficult to establish.

Gene-mutation, which may by itself be lethal and is certainly important for the cell involved, has also been regarded since the classic work of Müller as a one-hit process for which there was no recovery. Recent work stemming from the mouse geneticists at Oak Ridge and Harwell and from microbiological investigations now throws doubt on the universal validity of this concept. For certain germ cells, such as spermatogonia, the mutation-rate induced by a given dose of X-rays depends to a measurable extent on the dose-rate at which the irradiation was given and the age of the mouse. Presumably, as with bacteria, the metabolic state of the cells is of some consequence.

RADIOTOXICITY IN PERSPECTIVE

I have adopted so far the more or less classical and historical approach to radio-intoxication. Interest in the biological effects of radiation grew out of applying radiation for treatment, that is for destruction of unwanted growths. It meant the utilization of the brute force of radiation with large doses and usually at high intensities. The experimental work has therefore been mainly with large doses and high dose-rates. The consequential biological effects are severe.

In the world today radiation is playing an increasing role in medical treatment, so the better understanding of all its biological effects is necessary. Moreover, the information is directly relevant to occupational work with atomic energy under conditions of accident. Already the score of radiation casualties from reactor accidents is mounting in absolute numbers, though in relative terms, compared with other major industrial processes, atomic energy has produced remarkably few serious accidents. It is only too obvious that in circumstances of nuclear war radiation-casualties would pose a tremendous problem. However, most of our thinking is in making radiation at profoundly lower levels safe to live with.

Hitherto where I have mentioned doses of radiation, these have been measured by the thousands of units—rads. This is the radiotherapeutic range, and for X-rays these doses are given at intensities of ten or even hundreds of rads per minute. At the opposite end of the scale we have to consider natural background radiation, where the dose-rate is relatively uniform and extremely low, averaging about one-tenth of a rad per year in tissue. These intensities may have some biological effect: in fact theory demands that this should not be zero. Nevertheless we must be clear that no such effect has yet been measured.

Between these two extremes is the zone of interest. Those occupationally employed with radiations are permitted under present regulations to accumulate up to 200 rads of γ-rays, or the equivalent in other radiations, during the course of a working lifetime. They are under constant physical and medical surveillance. Members of the public, who are not under control in this way, are limited by regulation to intensities of irradiation some thirty times lower. These regulations have been based on past experience in radiology and on calculations based on experiments. The principle is that permissible values are some ten times lower than anything experience or experiment has shown to be deleterious. Note that theory predicts that, in so far as some effects of radiations, for example mutations in certain cells, are produced in direct proportion to radiation-dose irrespective of intensity, these values are not zero, just as they presumably are not zero for natural background radiation. The philosophy is that by doubling or even trebling the radiation-dose from natural background the effects should not be demonstrable. Certain localized areas in the world which support life apparently with complete success have a natural background which is up to ten times the average for the world at large.

The object of all experiment, therefore, is to record observations at levels of dose or intensity where statistically significant results can be obtained and thereby to make existing theory more precise or to act as foundations for new theory. The ultimate hope would be to check the theory by experiment at the levels of interest down to natural background. The prospects of this being accomplished in our time are remote.

This exposition should give us some of the picture. However, it is meet to contrast radiation hazards in general with some others.

Frequently one is given a comparison with the "toll of the roads" due to automobiles and similar mechanical devices of the present century. In the United Kingdom more than 5,000 people are killed on the roads each year, and many times more are injured. Some of us smugly say how incomparably smaller are the numbers of injuries from radiation. The analogy, however, is not necessarily exact. Deaths "on the road" can be patently referred to a particular incident: they are deaths from violence and not, in legal jargon, from natural causes. Deaths and injuries from certain reactor accidents and the like may be comparable: but the sequelae of other radiation injuries from occupational exposure, natural background, or fallout, in descending order of contribution to tissue-dose in the individual at the time of writing, would find expression ultimately, perhaps after scores of years, as natural causes.

RESPONSE TO RADIOTOXIC EFFECT

In a complex organism such as the mammal, the response in the various tissues is limited. Some or all of the cells may apparently be completely unaffected. This does not exclude the possibility that some permanent damage has been done and that our present methods of investigation are too crude to detect the lesion.

Death of cells may occur as has been described. If, as for nerve cells and perhaps oöcytes, a mechanism for replacement does not exist, the functional damage is permanent. The physical space left by death of cells en masse is often replaced by scar tissue. This is what occurs, for example, in a cardiac infarct following coronary thrombosis; the surviving cells then undergo hypertrophy in response to the additional fractional load placed on them. Alternatively, if there is a mechanism for replacement, the existing cells can by multiplication fill the physical space vacated. This is the situation one expects for skin and bone marrow.

If the damage is less than lethal, affected cells may undergo degeneration but survive impaired. This may be recognizable in diminished function or anatomically as atrophy. Physiological atrophy occurs from disuse or interference with supply of blood and nutrients—it is reversible when the cause is removed. The reason for all atrophy is not yet determined, notably the atrophy of old age.

Undifferentiated cells, which provide a pool from which the requisite number in unit time are withdrawn for maturation, may react to injury by differentiation. This might be considered as a normal change, prematurely induced. If the residual undifferentiated cells can divide to refill the pool, continuity of the stock is insured. Lajtha(8) has presented arguments indicating that this is the normal mechanism in maintaining the cellularity of bone marrow and that refilling of the pool of primitive cells occurs after depletion by ionizing radiation. On the other hand, if the number of primitive cells in the pool is fixed, as it is for oöcytes, any premature differentiation would mean a shortening of the functional life of the organ.

In contrast to this normal change, abnormal change or malignant transformation to cancer can occur. While we recognize now a large number of cancer-inducing agents, chemical and physical, we would not continue to be spending so much money on cancer research if we understood what malignant transformation really was.

The social problems of this century in countries of advanced civilization are now different from those in the same countries in previous eras or in countries of primitive standard today. The lethal factors under these latter conditions are infection with viruses, bacteria, and primitive organisms. This is Nature's biological warfare directed against itself. We have learned to defend ourselves and our biological sources of food against this attack and to survive on the average for three-score years and ten. We have lengthened enormously the average life span but not one whit the maximum life span. We are up against new problems for solution, the conquest of the degenerative and malignant diseases. To provide the best defense against these, which may be likened to Nature's chemical and radiological weapons, we have got to have a good understanding of the natural histories of the diseases they induce. This may well be more difficult than with infections, many of which are blitzkriegs and most of which have early manifestations. But the attacks by natural chemical and radiological noxa are much more insidious and cumulative. Furthermore there are natural defenses against infecting organisms—the study of them is the science of immunology—but we have as yet little knowledge of what natural allies we have against the agents which cause the shades of the mortuary to close around the growing boy.

References

1. BERGONIÉ, J., and TRIBONDEAU, L. Translation from C. R. Acad. Sci., 143: 983. 1906. *In:* Radiat. Res., 11: 587. 1959.
2. STOCKEN, L. A. Radiat. Res., Supp. 1, 53. 1959.
3. TROWELL, O. A. Internat. J. Rad. Biol., 4: 163. 1961.
4. OAKBERG, E. F. J. Exp. Zool., 134: 343. 1957.
5. ALEXANDER, P. Atomic Radiation and Life. Penguin Books, London. 1957.
6. BRUES, A. M. Science, 128: 793. 1958.
7. TOUGH, I.; COURT BROWN, W. M.; BAIKIE, A. G.; BUCKTON, K.; HARNDEN, D. G.; JACOBS, P.; KING, M.; and McBRIDE, J. A. Lancet, 1: 411. 1961.
8. LAJTHA, L. G., and OLIVER, R. *In:* Haemopoiesis, CIBA Foundation Symposium, p. 289. J. & A. Churchill, London. 1960.

CHAPTER TWO

CANCER, LEUKEMIA, AND LONGEVITY

Life Span

NATURAL AGING

Once upon a time there was a varied but recurrent advertisement for a well-known brand of cigarettes with the title: "Nature in the raw is seldom mild." This is a statement of a well-known truth as far as living things are concerned. In the competition for available nutrients only the strongest and biologically fittest survive. Trees, it is true, may live to a very venerable age, but in the zoölogical world longevity under natural conditions is not the norm. Once the individual has passed the peak for his particular genus his chances of survival in a competitive world are poor. There are few problems of senescence, therefore, in nature.

Man has risen above this level owing to the march of civilization. However, even for Man senescence has been of minor sociological importance till recently, though we are only too well aware of it as a factor in the present century. In the past what controlled the size and age distribution of human populations were wars and pestilence, and of these the more puissant was pestilence. Where deaths in war were measured by the thousands, loss of life by disease accounted for millions. A century of improvement in hygiene and a half century's accumulation of knowledge of bacteriology, microbiology, and immunology has completely altered that. Epidemics and pandemics due to infection and infestation can now be controlled. The average life span of a human population of an advanced degree of civilization is thus three-score years and ten, plus a year or two for women, minus a year or two for men. Notably, the maximum life span has not altered. We can discount the 969 years of Methuselah and accept that one hundred years, plus a little, is the maximum now and was in the past.

What has happened is that one threshold has been crossed, the conquest of infections, and we are up against another, senescence. We must be honest and say that at the present time we know about as much of the fundamentals of this problem as our eighteenth-century ancestors with their primitive microscopes knew about germs. Pessimists will say that this threshold will never be crossed, that we are now asked to prevent the ravages of fair wear and tear. Optimists will remain optimists and compare the living system with the engineer's hardware, speculating on the possibilities of reducing wear and of replacing damaged parts.

Leaving speculation aside we can study life tables to see why people die, for instance, in the United Kingdom or the U.S.A. The preponderant causes of death can be summed into two classes— degenerative diseases, particularly of the cardiovascular system, and cancer. In some of the circles in which I move these two classes are considered apart and one talks of the "problem of aging" and the "problem of cancer." This may be convenient for budgetary purposes and even for pathological classification, but basically both classes have the common feature of time. The probability of an individual's dying of cancer increases according to a high power (>2) of his age (1, 2). Even those that die at great ages of degenerative diseases are usually veritable museums of tumors, mostly benign but some malignant. Thus the terminal event which determines the certified cause of death may be largely a matter of chance. In the same way those that die at great ages of cancer have a miscellany of degenerations in various tissues, some of which by act of God could have "failed" with lethal results.

There has been much written about life and theories of life that I have not read. I can, however, quote bits from here and there.

A most able authority (3) from Chicago states: "Death is a physiological event and must be understood in its dependence on the physiological state of the organism. . . . A theory that fits the physiological facts states that death is a random event arising from an extreme fluctuation of the physiological state of the individual." I would quarrel with some of the uses of the adjective "physiological" here, but, that aside, the thesis propounded is that life is a matter of random ups and downs, one of which happens to exceed a critical value and that is death. This is quite at variance with my idea of the physiological state, which is one of wheels within wheels to preserve a steady state, a series of compensatory mechanisms, feedbacks, and adjustments to avoid extreme fluctuation. Failure of a compensatory mechanism may certainly lead to a swing in one direction, but such failure is a matter of disease, that is a pathological not a physiological state.

However, the concept of a randomness of mortality is extremely widely held. It may be tantamount to saying that the environment with its various stresses results in strains which summate to cause death. Alternatively it can be invoked as mutation or similar process affecting the genetic background. My colleague, Neary (4), has summarized the situation about the contrasting theories of aging:

Random theories. Theories in this category, while recognizing that the outcome of the interaction between an environment and an individual depends on his genetic make-up, are concerned with the behaviour of a population of supposedly uniform individuals. Such theories attach considerable significance to the empirical age-specific death-rate, the so-called "force of mortality," sometimes interpreted as the probability per unit time that any survivor will die in that time interval. For this to be true in an exact quantitative sense, all the individuals alive at a given instant would have to be identical, a qualification pointed out by Medawar [5], but not always sufficiently noted. The fact that the force of mortality in most populations increases with age beyond a certain point has been accepted as evidence of a progressive change in the population with age. Gompertz [6] noted that in human populations the logarithm of the age-specific death rate increases approximately linearly with age from early maturity onwards, and so this quantity has been regarded as a general measure of physiological state, and its rate of change (approximately

constant) as a measure of the rate of physiological ageing of the population, and even by tacit assumption of each individual member thereof [7].
Sacher [8] has elaborated on these ideas in an elegant mathematical model
which assumes that the individuals in the population are initially identical,
but that due to random external stresses and physiological interactions
there is a progressive drift and dispersion in the physiological states of
these individuals. The death of an individual occurs when his physiological
state transcends a certain limit. In this model the logarithm of the age-
specific death-rate is directly proportional to the *mean* physiological state
of the population at that age; the empirical Gompertz relation would thus
seem to imply that the mean state changes linearly with time. The reality
of the rate of physiological ageing so deduced will depend in any actual
situation on the validity, among other things, of the assumption of initial
identity of all individuals.

A progressive decline in physiological state or vitality is thus an essential feature of theories assuming random mortality, but a detailed causative mechanism for the decline itself is not usually specified.

Genetically determinate theories. These theories concentrate attention
on the individual rather than the population and, in their quantitative
aspects at least, on the component cells of the individual. The environment
is scarcely considered explicitly, except as a more or less uniform influence;
for a given environment the life-span of the individual is predetermined
by the initial genetic endowment. In some theories, ageing is regarded as
some process of change within cells themselves, possibly in their genetic
apparatus (9—13). . . . but it is clear at once that the fate of the individual cannot be considered solely in terms of the fate of a component
cell. In an animal, the cells are organized in a complex hierarchy of inter-
acting anatomical and physiological systems. Thus while changes within
cells may be the root cause of ageing and finally death, it may be appropriate to consider the whole sequence of events solely in terms of the
primary process.

It should be fairly clear that in nature the genetic background
and the environment both play a part. In the laboratory we are
able to control some of the factors which are variable in nature.

The genetic constitution of animals, which in nature leads to
variety in form and function, can be made less variable by prolonged inbreeding. Usually this results in a diminished vigor of the
stock, but in some species, and notably mice among mammals,
selected strains can be developed which are quite hardy in the

environment of the laboratory. In fact many strains of mice have been strictly inbred by brother-sister mating for scores of generations. This results in stocks which are extremely (but never absolutely) homogeneous. Such stocks were developed for many laboratory purposes; they can be used for longevity studies to overcome the genetic variability inherent in wild-type stocks.

Environmental factors can also be standardized to a considerable extent. By some soft-hearted "animal-lovers," the life of the laboratory animal is depicted as one of pain and misery. On the contrary, for the majority it is one of idleness, leisure, abundance of food and drink, and protection against natural predators. It could be argued that far more often than otherwise the experimenter is pampering his animals and "killing them by kindness." Some environmental hazards, however, still remain. Mice, for instance, may still fight among themselves even when food is superabundant and sexual rivalry is not involved. This can be overcome at the expense of individual caging and presumably boredom. Natural disease is another problem. As with human populations the infective diseases can be reduced to a minimum by scrupulous attention to hygiene, and this is practiced by all reputable experimenters. A system of quarantine is also observed in the case of all new entrants to the animal house. In spite of all these precautions some bacterial infections may occur, and we are becoming increasingly aware of the role of viruses, not only in diseases which have long been recognized as infective, for example, hepatitis, but also in cancer. Some of these viruses are naturally endemic in the stocks and may be passed from generation to generation by the usual contacts and even in the germ plasm or in the maternal milk from mother to offspring.

Given these limitations, useful work in the laboratory can be carried out on longevity. In the past most of the effort has gone into study of the natural history of cancers. Particularly in the last decade, however, some have been turning their attention to the other phenomena of aging animals. The stimulus for this has come from the social consequences of increased longevity with the increasing role of geriatrics in medical practice and on the other hand from the fears of a reversal of the former trend in average longevity as a result of radiations from the "new atomic age."

RADIATION AND AGING

Ionizing radiations have been recognized since the discovery of X-rays by Roentgen and of radioactivity by Becquerel in the closing years of the last century. The application of X-rays to medical diagnosis was immediately obvious, though, as Spear (14) describes,

the fact that living tissues may be damaged by the passage of X-rays through them was only recognized later.

There are two main reasons for this: firstly the relatively small amount of radiation required to produce an X-ray shadow compared with the very large dose which is required to produce any immediately recognizable biological change; and secondly the time interval (now called the "latent period") which elapses between ordinary exposures and the appearance of any visible biological reaction. As a consequence enthusiastic roentgenologists repeatedly cast shadows of their hands upon fluorescent screens heedless of the accompanying useless rays (the long wavelength or "soft" radiation) which were unwittingly being absorbed in excessive amounts by the surface layers of the skin exposed to the unprotected X-ray tube. These rays contributed nothing to the casting of the shadow though in the aggregate they led to significant biological changes. Even longer exposures were needed to produce X-ray photographs of which Röntgen himself took the first; though he, by keeping his tube in a box, obtained protection from the most damaging rays which some others, using the uncovered tube, lacked. When skin troubles eventually appeared, as they did in quite early days, they were at first "explained away" on other grounds than X-ray damage and so the mischief went on.

When the damaging action of X-rays on tissue was confirmed, the rays were logically applied for their destructive action on unwanted tissues such as cancers and, because of their observed action on skin, somewhat less logically, to all manner of skin diseases. To quote Spear (14) again: "Any evidence of a beneficial effect of radiation was hailed with delight; accidents were neglected and the lessons they should have taught disregarded until the number of tragedies began to mount to alarming proportions. . . . It is estimated that by 1922 one hundred radiologists had died from malignant disease due to radiation." In other words an occupational hazard was established.

The story of radium was much the same. The Curies, working with large quantities of ores of uranium, which Becquerel had shown to fog photographic plate through its wrappings, were able to separate two new elements, radium and polonium, which were highly radioactive. Radium is long-lived (half-life ~5,000 years) and itself emits the poorly penetrating α-rays; but it decays through a series of daughter elements some of which emit β- and γ-rays. The first decay product is the noble gas, radon, which readily escapes, but if radium is kept in sealed containers the radon is preserved and decays *in situ* with a half-life of a few days rapidly through very short-lived daughters (RaA, RaB, RaC, RaC'), which provide much of the β, γ emission, to 22-year RaD, an isotope of lead. The walls of the sealed containers absorb all of the α-rays and usually by design all of the β-rays too. Thus sealed quantities of radium can be utilized as sources of γ-rays—and like X-rays these have been widely used in medical therapy—but historically, as Spear (14) points out, by a different group of practitioners from the purveyors of X-rays. The linking of X-ray and radium work is a relatively modern innovation.

The radium surgeons did derive some protection against the superficially damaging β-rays and from the fact that their sources were sealed. The chemists who purified the radium and the technicians who prepared sources were not so fortunate. They were not only exposed to the external γ-irradiation but, in their ignorance of the hazards of even trace quantities of these materials, in air to be respired or on fingers to be wittingly or unwittingly licked, allowed their bodies to become contaminated. In the tissues, notably the bones, there was no capsule to absorb the very energetic and locally damaging α- and β-rays.

Thus more occupational hazards in a variety of trades and professions associated with radium were ultimately recognized. Perhaps the most notorious was the uncovering after World War I of the dangers of luminizing—applying radioactive paint to watches, instruments, etc. The luminizers, mostly young girls at the time

of employment, suffered from severe and often fatal anemia due to
the irradiation of their blood-forming bone marrow from radioactive materials deposited in their bones, if their corporeal contamination was large—and by large one means the very small
amount in absolute terms of 10–100 μg. of radium; with smaller
burdens of 1–10 μg. of radium, the limiting danger was due to
death of bone cells (necrosis) or to malignant transformation,
osteosarcoma.

These were the occupational problems of radiation in the first
three decades of the present century. A similar problem had
existed for centuries—for example, as the cause of lung cancer in
miners of the Schneeberg in Saxony and nearby regions of Bohemia
—but radiation was incriminated only in the twentieth. These
mines, which are rich in a variety of ores, are now a commercial
source of uranium. In the chain of decay from uranium down to
radium and beyond, the gas radon is released and with inadequate
ventilation can reach relatively high values in mines. The short-
lived decay products of the radon are adsorbed onto dust which is
plentiful everywhere and especially in mines. Each dust particle
has a high probability of being trapped on inspiration somewhere
in the respiratory tract, where it can release its energy on disinte-
gration of its radioactive load.

There is little question that, on the whole, occupations of the
past involving ionizing radiation and radioactivity have been
associated with premature deaths of workers, mainly due to
malignant disease. It is very difficult and at best rather speculative
to attempt to describe these death rates in conventional and
acceptable quantitative terms.

It is noteworthy, however, that the malignancies of this recent
era usually accepted as radiation-induced include skin cancers of
X-ray workers and manipulators of radium and radioactive materials, bronchial cancers of the miners, and bone cancers of the
luminizers. At the time leukemia—or malignant transformation
of the blood-forming tissues—was not incriminated. In retrospect
it is possible to make out a case for leukemia being a hazard from
certain forms of exposure to radiation (and a list of individuals

affected by the disease would include many well-known names of radiation pioneers) but leukemia does not seem to be similarly prominent when the causes of death of luminizers are scrutinized. What is not so certain is whether radiation workers of the past have suffered any loss of expected life span from other causes which can be aggregated under the term early senescence. A number of inquiring people have looked at the data available from the radiological profession.

The obituary notices of members of the medical profession published in the *Journal of the American Medical Association* have supplied much information. From this source March (15) identified leukemia as a prominent cause of death in radiologists, being listed about ten times more commonly than for non-radiological members of the profession. Members of the profession as a whole were more commonly affected than their non-medical counterparts in the general population according to Henshaw and Hawkins (16) and Dublin and Spiegelman (17), but March regarded this as largely due to the radiologists in the profession.

From the same source Shields Warren (18) collected information for a period of 25 years on 82,441 deaths, noting not only cause of death where reported but age at death. From the data it appeared that the average age at death of radiologists was 60.5 years against 62.3 for dermatologists and 63.7 for certain other specialists with some contact with radiation, and 65.7 for all physicians and 65.6 for white males in the U.S.A. It appeared also that radiologists died younger than the other groups not only from leukemia but from practically every cause of death. Thus it seemed that the aging process was hastened by their occupation.

Warren had realized that the age structure of radiologists was a factor to be reckoned with and had compared it with that of pathologists, another specialty, finding no significant difference. Later, however, a further look at this factor was taken by Seltser and Sartwell (19), who found radiologists in the U.S.A. to be a younger group in general than the profession at large. If Warren's data are corrected for the age structure of radiologists, their premature demise is no longer apparent.

In the United Kingdom Court Brown and Doll (20) examined the mortality of 1,377 British radiologists and arrived at the following conclusions:

1. A study of the mortality of British radiologists during the period 1897 to 1956 reveals no evidence of any non-specific reduction in their life expectancy, such as could be provided by an increase in the age-specific mortality rates for all causes of death.

2. There is evidence amongst those entering radiological practice prior to 1921 of an increased mortality rate from skin cancer, an unexpected increased mortality from tumours of the pancreas, the significance of which can only be assessed after further data have been obtained on pancreatic sensitivity, and a very small increase in mortality from leukaemia.

3. British radiologists who have started radiology since 1920 may well not have incurred any appreciable hazard. It must be borne in mind, however, that the induction periods for radiation-induced tumours may be 20 years or more and final judgement of the efficiency of protective measures must await the outcome of a longer period of observation. The findings do suggest, however, that provided care is taken to introduce and observe reasonable measures of protection, the long-term somatic risks of irradiation will be very small.

Thus in spite of what we know now about the biological hazards of radiation and how before 1921 precautions were virtually non-existent, we can find in small populations practicing in those days no overt signs of non-specific aging, though we can identify some induction of malignancy.

Many imponderables have to be mentioned. We do not know the effective doses of radiation received by the practitioners of those days. We do know that, compared with today's, their apparatus was primitive. Historical relics can be made to function again, and the exposures derived from them at various distances measured; but we can only estimate roughly the total exposure times and places of radiologists. We do know that these sets were of considerably lower voltage than those in use today, so that radiations received by the body from them were much less penetrating. Hence the predominance of skin lesions and cancers among observed effects. Whereas the skin of hands of the previous generations of practitioners may have been exposed to over 1,000 roentgens, the dose in deep tissues was relatively greatly reduced. We know also from the nature of the work that the dosage was intermittent and of high dose-rate when the dose was applied, conditions which we now know to be more productive of certain malignant changes than the same total dosage uniformly given in time at low dose-rate; but we do not know much about the relation of dosage schedules to induction of degenerative lesions.

Experimental Studies

To supplement the clinical and epidemiological observations, there has naturally been recourse to experimental studies with animals. In general these can be divided into two classes, those in which groups of animals are given single doses of ionizing radiation of different sizes and then followed for the development of delayed lesions attributable to that insult, and those in which groups of animals are kept permanently in radiation fields of different intensity from a fixed time in their life history, usually early, until their death.

SINGLE DOSES

The life-shortening effects of single doses of radiation given to mice and rats were illustrated by the United Nations Scientific Committee on the Effects of Atomic Radiation (21) (Fig. 12). The linear relation between effect and dose suggests that one could calculate the life-shortening to be expected from each unit of radiation, e.g. rem. However, as the Committee were careful to point out, this relation pertains only to rather intense radiation—at lower dose-rates different numerical values would be obtained; moreover, it applies only when the whole body is exposed—partial exposure greatly modifies the result; and it applies only to adolescent animals.

Since the U.N. Committee issued its first report, the results of a large experiment of this sort in the United Kingdom have become available. In the inbred mice used by Lindop and Rotblat (22, 23)

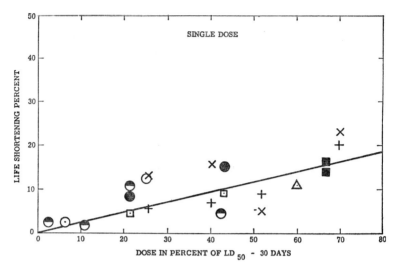

FIG. 12.—Life shortening (percentage) in mice and rats after a single whole-body exposure to X- or γ-rays. The dose is expressed as a percentage of the acute LD 50. (From United Nations Scientific Committee, *Report on the Effects of Atomic Radiation* [New York, 1958] Fig. 3, Annex G).

the reduction in life span was, as classical, proportional to dose. The Gompertz plots of specific death rate versus age were not linear. Empirically a linear relation was found between probit of percentage mortality versus the square of age at death (Fig. 13). Having noted that they had given whole body irradiation of high intensity at probably the most sensitive stage of the mouse's life (4 weeks) the authors state:

> The fact that the corrected survival curves are parallel to each other after the "plateau" region, suggests that life shortening is the result of a loss of a few weeks of early life and not of a contraction of the time scale of the animal's life. From the point of view of survival the irradiated mice behave exactly like their non-irradiated mates of an older age and only in this sense can one claim that radiation causes premature ageing by an amount proportional to the dose.

While the numerical data are valuable in that they provide confirmatory evidence of former studies, the supplementary analysis of causes of death is still more illuminating because of the general paucity of information on the pathological side.

While all causes of death were advanced by radiation some were advanced faster than others: in particular leukaemia was advanced more and pulmonary tumours less than the average. . . . In this investigation, in which the irradiation was given at the age of 30 days, when the haemopoietic tissue is most active, leukaemia was most advanced by radiation. Exposure at another age may well bring to the fore a completely different disease.

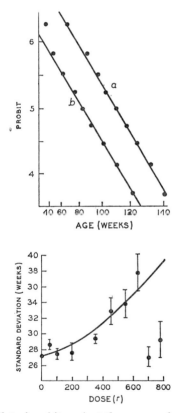

Fig. 13.—*Top*: Plot of probit against the square of age for mice of both sexes; *a*, control group; *b*, 457 r group. *Bottom*: Standard deviation of distribution of ages at death as a function of dose. (From P. Lindop and J. Rotblat, *Proc. Roy. Soc.*, Ser. B, 154: 332, 350, Figs. 7, 8.)

CHRONIC DOSAGE

The conventional dose-rate for single doses of some tens or hundreds of roentgens is about 50 r/min. The dose-rate of Lindop and Rotblat was 500 r/min. A factor of 10 in either direction from 50 r/min is not likely on standard radiobiological theory to cause any great difference in effect, and, if one believes that biological observations made on mice and rats can be transposed to men, then the situation, as far as dose-rate is concerned, is comparable with certain occupational accidents, for example, reactor excursions.

However, we are also concerned with increased contamination of the environment with radioactive materials from military or civil operations, which would raise the background of exposure to ionizing radiation. The natural background of radiation from cosmic and terrestrial sources is given as around 100 milliroentgens a year, though a few inhabited localities, because of altitude or geological formation, may have backgrounds greater by up to 10 times or so. These dose-rates are some 100 million times less than what was being considered in the previous section. It is natural, therefore, that experimenters should have taken the alternative course and exposed animals to dose-rates of radiation which approximate more to the foreseeable conditions of environmental contamination.

Young animals which are placed in a radiation field, usually produced by sources of natural radium or man-made cobalt 60 or cesium 137, and kept there for the rest of their lives may accumulate doses of many thousands of rads before they die. Given at a high dose-rate these doses would be lethal within a few days. It is therefore conventional to talk of recovery by certain tissues (see chap. i and yet to presume that there might be additional effects of a given dose from which there is no recovery. With chronic radiation these irrecoverable fractions should summate and lead to recognizable effects.

The results of a number of such experiments were also reviewed by the United Nations Scientific Committee, which quoted an assessment made by my colleague R. H. Mole (24). Both for γ-rays and for fast neutrons for which a relative biological effectiveness (RBE) of 13 compared with γ-rays was calculated, dose-rates which provided less than 10 r or equivalent per week did not significantly shorten the life span of the animals (Fig. 14). As Mole

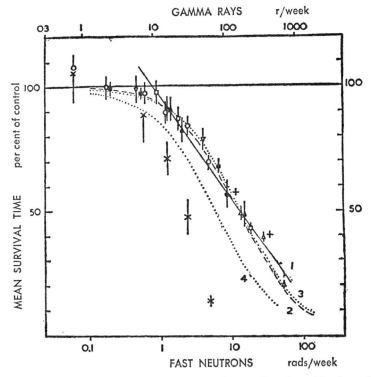

FIG. 14.—Mean survival time (per cent of control) and weekly dose of radiation (logarithmic scale). The gamma and neutron scales are in the ratio 13: 1. (From United Nations Scientific Committee, *Report on the Effects of Atomic Radiation* [New York, 1958], Annex G.)

pointed out, the observations were compatible both with the concept of an incremental effect for each unit of dose and with a "threshold" of dose-rate necessary to produce an effect. The threshold could be either absolute or relative, that is in the latter case needing so long for development that the animal would have died before the effect was manifest.

The whole question of thresholds is a very thorny one and the following is a balanced view from the Medical Research Council's *Hazards to Man of Nuclear and Allied Radiations* (1960 [25]):

> The use of the term "threshold" is based on the concept that for particular forms of radiation damage a minimum dose can be established below which no effect will be produced. This term, however, involves oversimplifications which can be very misleading.
>
> Any radiation exposure is likely to produce some changes in at least a few cells, although the normal processes of tissue repair may be adequate to reverse these changes if they are very slight or if they are caused at a very slow rate. The essential difficulty is to decide whether an apparent threshold is due to a genuine absence of effect at low doses or to a failure to observe the effect owing to the very low frequency at which it is occurring. It might be due to the latter if the frequency with which an effect occurred were directly proportional to the dose received, but would be even more likely to be so if this frequency were proportional to the square of the dose or to some other power.
>
> There are great practical difficulties in planning any investigation to decide this issue. The probability of the occurrence of harmful effects following low doses may be so small, or the delay in their induction so prolonged, as to make it impossible to design a sufficiently extensive study to demonstrate them. This difficulty applies particularly to the investigation of the effects on man of low doses received at a slow rate like the radiation from the natural background or from artificial sources such as fall-out which give even smaller rates.
>
> On the other hand, it is often possible to study the effects of a considerable range of moderate and larger doses. If, however, at these doses a certain effect is found to be proportional to the dose received, it is not necessarily justifiable to infer that the same relationship would hold at lower doses or to conclude that a threshold did not exist at some dose below those studied.
>
> In any case, the concept of a single "threshold" dose applicable to all circumstances can hardly be valid since sensitivity to radiation may vary according to many factors including the tissue irradiated, the age of the individual, the type of radiation and pattern of dosage. What we need to know in any set of circumstances is the frequency with which a particular form of adverse effect is caused by different doses of radiation and the way in which the likelihood of such effects increases as the dose of radiation increases.
>
> Although we have now sufficient knowledge to make an approximate assessment of the damage to be expected from high and moderate rates

of radiation exposure, we can at present only infer the degree of damage likely to be caused by low rates of exposure. In considering the possible practical effects on man of exposure to radiation, we therefore think it prudent to continue to assume that even the lowest doses of radiation may involve a finite, though correspondingly low, probability of adverse effect. This may prove to be an unduly cautious estimate but, in our opinion, it is only the justifiable one in the present state of our knowledge.

This is a careful opinion stated in the language of the scientist. In life outside the laboratory other judgments, social, political, and moral, have to be weighed with the scientific. In this instance a number of workers in different laboratories have shown that with the numbers of animals available to them no difference in longevity is discernible between the unirradiated and those irradiated up to 10 r per week. A real difference of 10 per cent could certainly, and one of 5 per cent would probably, have been determined with the numbers of animals used. The value judgment of a scientific body like the International Commission on Radiological Protection (26) is

to limit the radiation dose to that which involves a risk that is not unacceptable to the individual and to the population at large. This is called a "permissible dose."

The permissible dose for an individual is that dose, accumulated over a long period of time or resulting from a single exposure, which, in the light of present knowledge, causes a negligible probability of severe somatic or genetic injuries; furthermore it is such a dose that any effects that ensue more frequently are limited to those of a minor nature that would not be considered unacceptable by the exposed individual or by competent medical authorities.

This judgment by a scientific body which has attempted to weigh the disadvantages of exposure to ionizing radiations against the benefits from medical and industrial applications of the same radiations has not been seriously challenged by the social, political, legal, or religious bodies. Any dissent is in the quantitation of where to draw the line.

In terms of somatic effects of radiations, the maintenance of a normal life span is probably as good a general guide as any, for it is a measure of the sum of all serious disabilities. The permissible dose for the occupational worker is now reckoned by the International Commission as an average of 5 r per year for a working life of 40 years. This is possibly some ten times less than what radiologists of the past generation received with results that have been reviewed above. It is some one hundred times less than what has been shown to be a limiting value for populations of some hundreds of mice before they exhibit significant shortening of life span.

The question frequently asked by those who attach considerable weight to results of animal experiments is why not extend the numbers of animals used in the experiment from hundreds to hundreds of thousands. The quick answer is of course the great cost. The best answer, however, is that such an experiment under ideal conditions would improve the precision of results by the square root of the numbers of animals involved—that is a law of diminishing returns operates. More important, conditions are never ideal. In a small experiment there can be uniformity of environment, supervision, and interpretation. Beyond a certain point this cannot be maintained. Thus to enlarge the numbers would mean the introduction of other rather poorly controlled variables. The final result would be no real increase in precision, which is the object of the exercise.

In circumstances such as these, the conventional procedure is to argue: Instead of proceeding by bulldozing tactics, let us try to learn about fundamental mechanisms on which we can build a superstructure by calculation. This is an admirable principle, but while it is easy (but unpopular) to instruct staff to undertake a frontal attack with bulldozers, it is not easy to do the outflanking maneuver without losing the way. Only the really great can uncover the right fundamental information to order. Lesser lights assemble apparently irrelevant observations of others and develop them to make meaning in contexts hitherto unsuspected. Ordinary research workers just discover things, the lucky ones being those who discover things which are obviously important or of which brighter boys can see the importance.

There may well be enough existing fundamental information for a working understanding of malignant transformation and senescence. Suffice it to say that none of the masters has assembled and presented it in such a way as to gain universal acceptance. Thus ordinary mortals go on collecting observations by direct and indirect means.

In my own laboratory Neary (4) and Mole (24) with their respective colleagues, following a first experiment which took 3 years to complete and a similar period to collate and interpret, have continued to expose groups of animals to chronic irradiation from both γ-rays of cobalt 60 and fast neutrons. One problem for solution is, "Does chronic irradiation, which reduces the mean life span according to the mean accumulated dose, do so by accelerating the processes of aging?" In this case the cumulative mortality curve of an irradiated group would be like that of the unirradiated with the time axis contracted, and the dispersion of lifetimes in the irradiated group would be reduced in proportion to the mean

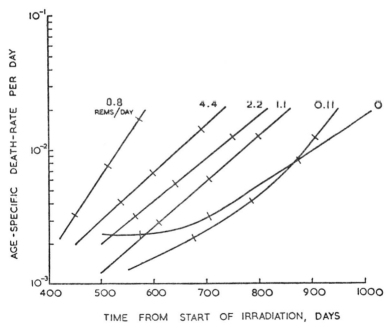

FIG. 15.—Gompertz plots, LAF$_1$ mice, males and females combined. (From G. J. Neary, in *Nature* [Lond.], 187: 10.)

lifetime. In the classical experiments of Lorenz *et al.* (28) with
LAF₁ mice, this was approximately so (Fig. 15), but not in the
CBA mice of our laboratory (Figs. 16 and 17). There the cumula-
tive mortality of the irradiated group corresponded to that of
unirradiated with the time axis displaced but not contracted.
Thus Neary, Munson, and Mole (27) postulate premature aging

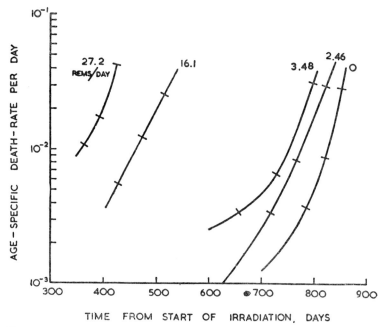

FIG. 16.—Gompertz plots, CBA mice, males. (From G. J. Neary, in
Nature [Lond.], **187:** 10, Fig. 3.)

rather than accelerated aging—and this is the conclusion of Lindop
and Rotblat (22) for single doses of high-intensity radiation.

To explain "premature aging" Neary (4) considers aging
as a two-stage process, induction and development. The second
stage is roughly constant in length, some six months in the mouse,
but the inductive phase, which would be of variable length in different strains according to genetical background, can be shortened
by artifice, for example, by irradiation or by a number of chemical

and infective agents. Jones (29) in an impressive monograph would allow all these noxious influences to summate. Thus Neary (4) envisages that "when such mice are chronically irradiated all individuals receive the same accumulated *effective* dose and all suffer the same shortening of the induction period."

In the quotation above, the adjective *effective* has been italicized

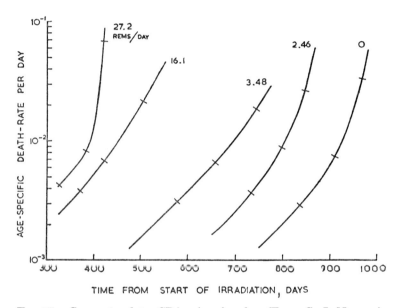

FIG. 17.—Gompertz plots, CBA mice, females. (From G. J. Neary, in *Nature* [Lond.], **187**: 10, Fig. 4.)

and with purpose. As Mole (30) pointed out at a comparatively early stage, in chronic irradiations of this kind much of the radiation must be wasted, notably that given in the terminal stages of the mouse's life in the radiation field. What would happen if the experimental animals were removed from the radiation field to normal surroundings after a limited period of exposure? If the later doses of continuous irradiation throughout life are indeed wasted, a limited exposure should be as effective in shortening life as the complete exposure. And such is the experience of our labo-

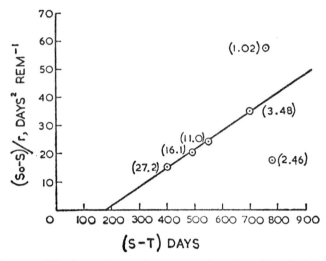

F<small>IG</small>. 18.—Life-shortening per dose-rate against time of irradiation. CBA mice, males. Numbers in brackets are daily dose-rates. The intercept is the mean development time. (From G. J. Neary, in *Nature* [Lond.], **187:** 10, Fig. 6.)

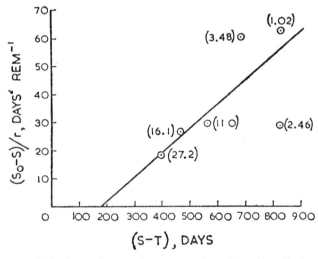

F<small>IG</small>. 19.—Life-shortening per dose-rate against time of irradiation. CBA mice, females. Numbers in brackets are daily dose-rates. The intercept is the mean development time. (From G. J. Neary, in *Nature* [Lond.], **187:** 10, Fig. 7.)

ratory to date (see Fig. 20). The mean accumulated dose to death for a group of animals or the accumulated dose for an individual can thus be misleading. Neary in fact finds that the developmental period D is about 6 months for CBA mice and this is shown in Figures 18 and 19, which graph the shortening of life $(S_0 - S$ days) per various dose-rates of radiation (rem/day) against days of irradiation $(S - T)$, T being the age at which mice enter the area.

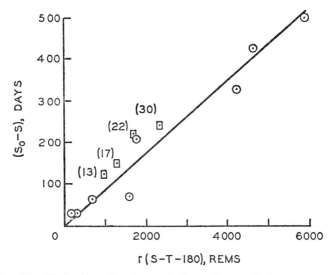

FIG. 20.—CBA mice, females. Life-shortening against mean accumulated effective dose. ⊙, lifetime irradiation; ⊡, irradiation for limited periods of weeks shown in brackets. (From G. J. Neary, in *Nature* [Lond.], **187**: 10, Fig. 9.)

For the effective dose, therefore, Neary takes that accumulated during the inductive period only, $r (S - T - D)$ of Figure 20.

The linear relation of shortening of life according to effective accumulated dose is compatible with the concept of a cumulative injury due to irreversible changes. In so far as this general relation holds for single doses of radiation (*vide supra*), for continuous irradiation from early life in limited periods and to death, and for a number of instances of fractionated doses, it is a wonderful boon to the planner. Administration is good only when it is simple. It is also prima facie favorable evidence for those who try to explain most of the phenomena of aging and malignant transformation in terms of somatic mutation.

However, the slope of the linear relation is not necessarily the same in each case. The life-shortening effect of chronic γ- and fast neutron irradiation is similar, so that Neary and Mole can consider the two together with an appropriate factor for the relative biological effectiveness (RBE) of fast neutrons. But X-rays given at high intensity are some three times more productive of effect than low intensity γ-rays. This too is like the mutational effects on some germ cells, e.g., spermatogonia (31), the relation of mutation rate to dose being linear in each case but of different slope.

The administrative action becomes more complex if one has these different slopes. The mutational hypothesis too becomes difficult to substantiate when a factor of 13 for RBE for fast neutrons is involved, while it is to be expected if we invoke damage to some relatively gross structure like a chromosome, rather than to a molecular structure. Furthermore as Neary (4) following Strehler (7) points out, if mutation is invoked, it is much more inefficient radiation than any we know, for to double the natural effect requires 5,000 rads of low-intensity γ-radiation or 1,500 rads of high-intensity X-radiation. The doubling dose for most effects generally accepted as mutational is usually in the region of 50 rads.

Whereas it is our duty as scientists to explain natural phenomena, physical and biological, to the layman so that the right social action may be taken, we have to admit that we cannot yet propound immutable scientific laws for aging. It is my belief, expressed earlier, that studies in life span provide the best integration of the effects of normal stresses and of radiation in man and animals, but to look only at the magic number, age at death, could blind us to some essential facts. In using lifespan as an integrator, we have to accept that the stress we are investigating, in our case radiation, acts equally with normal stresses in causing the strains which lead to death. In justifying themselves, some of those interested in problems of radiation have fallen over backward to postulate that all natural aging is due to natural background radiation. There is of course no evidence for this, and this form of monomania just makes life more difficult for those who have to consider other noxious agents, natural or man made.

In any serious study of aging attributable to an extra-natural influence, it is, therefore, essential as a second stage to look at the causes of death. This is the practice in our laboratory, but in only a few of the reported studies has such a procedure been followed. Hence my previously expressed approval of Lindop and Rotblat. Similar encomia are due to Upton *et al.* (32) for their monumental study on mice exposed to radiation from an atomic bomb. One far-reaching conclusion of a general nature from this work was that "there is no evidence that the effects observed in this study differ from those that would have been produced by comparable radiations delivered at a high intensity from conventional laboratory sources." The scientific conclusions included:

> The shortening of life-span was not attributable to increased mortality from any specific cause but was correlated with premature onset of all diseases associated with natural senescence. Although the effects of radiation on the incidence and severity of diseases of old age varied markedly from one disease to another all diseases were advanced in onset to essentially the same extent by any one dose of radiation, with the exception of thymic lymphoma.

I would emphasize the final clause, the exception. Thymic lymphoma is a form of leukemia with typical expression in the mouse. It will crop up again in the discussion on leukemia. This malignant growth was a prominent killer in the experiments of Upton *et al.* where the radiation was a single dose given at high intensity and of Lorenz *et al.* (28) in the laboratory with chronic γ-rays of low intensity. Both groups used the hybrid, LAF_1. Experiments in our own laboratory, mainly with CBA mice given low-intensity irradiation, have not indicated any particular prominence of this cause of death. Nevertheless, the condition can readily be induced in mice of the CBA and, in fact, of any strain, if the optimal conditions of exposure are explored. Kaplan and his colleagues (33) defined this many years ago for the C57BL mouse. Mole (34) has done it for CBA. In general a number of fractions of moderate-sized doses of radiation at high intensity spaced at intervals of about a week will give the maximum yield, which may approximate closely to 100 per cent of exposed mice. Clearly then for a condition like this we can produce more or less leukemia at will by radiation. Yet it is not a specific radiation disease in as much as it occurs naturally in practically all stocks, though to a degree varying from a negligible proportion to nearly all members; its incidence can be raised by agents other than radiation; and, again, owing to the studies of Kaplan and his group (35), the incidence can be reduced. If we have to consider thymic lymphoma as a cause of death in irradiated mice, we must specify not only dose, but dose-rate and time, possibly over-all, and certainly radiation-free time between exposures.

If there is one identified exception to a general formulation, there are probably more unidentified which need to be uncovered. Both as confirmation of the general proposition and in the search for exceptions, careful scrutiny of cause of death is required. This may double or treble the labor of an already tedious and largely unrewarding grind, but that literally is *re*search.

Need lack of knowledge of the fundamental causes of all the ills to which man and mice are prone and which are possibly speeded up by radiation delay development of the uses of radiation? Not if we are to learn from history. Mole (36) in another place has argued thus:

> How much of the mechanism needs to be known before control is possible? Historically it is fair to say that in no single instance has successful control of an environmental hazard depended on previous knowledge of the cellular mechanism involved. The nature of the life-cycle of the malarial parasite in the human body and the relative importance of the different kinds of immunity in human tuberculosis are of academic interest but not of first importance in controlling or preventing malaria or infection with tuberculosis. Lead poisoning and dust diseases of the lungs became wholly preventable as soon as it was realised there was a specific causal agent which could be avoided but their cellular mechanisms are still obscure.

We still have enough knowledge of the biological effects of radiation to have a profound, possibly exaggerated, respect for it. The feature that stands out is that large single doses of high intensity or multiple doses of moderate size can have decidedly deleterious delayed effects both in man and animals and so should be prevented. There is a strong suspicion that all radiation has a component of cumulative irrecoverable injury of an uncertain nature, but, unless the cumulative total is substantial, its biological manifestation is not distinguishable, even by statistical appraisal of large numbers either in man or animals.

What I have not considered hitherto is an alternative view that radiation in small doses may even be beneficial. This must certainly have been an acceptable view half a century ago from the widespread use of radiation in the therapy of many conditions. Probably much of the work was uncritical.

The idea became heretical with the rise in recent decades of the genetical concept that radiation is mutagenic and that practically all mutations are unfavorable both in germ cells, which the geneticist can evaluate, and by implication in somatic cells, which do not ordinarily lend themselves to genetic investigation.

Nevertheless the possibility has been raised again (37). In a number of studies on the life span of animals exposed to chronic irradiation, some groups have been included for irradiation at or about the levels considered permissible for the occupationally exposed man. In some but not all (which includes the work in our own laboratory) these groups so far from having a decreased life span have lived longer on average than the controls. In some cases this prolongation of life is not statistically significant and the longest-lived individuals are to be found in the unirradiated group. The longer mean life of the minimally irradiated can be attributed to chance and the features of the experiment. In some instances, notably with rats (Carlson and Jackson, 1959 [38]), the prolongation of life compared with the unirradiated was statistically significant. Suggestions have been made that this is due to the stock having, like many, an endemic disease of infective origin which is held in check by the radiation. Certainly more data will be required before it can be accepted that irradiation with low doses or at low dose-rates is "a good thing."

If we adopt the currently conventional attitude that all doses of radiation no matter how small have some cumulative effect which is to the subject's disadvantage, are we in a position to estimate it quantitatively? I should argue no. In the first place, as indicated above, there are other difficulties of adding the effects on longevity of high-intensity X-rays and low-intensity γ-rays. Nevertheless, some have attempted it to produce a figure for life-shortening of man per rem of chronic γ-radiation dose received but not, let it be noted, based upon the human statistics of radiologists. Instead the method was (to use the jargon) by extrapolation from experiments with animals. My knowledge of dog Latin allows me to deduce the first meaning of extrapolation as "an extra polish." It is in this sense, presumably with reference to the crystal ball, that the term must have been used.

The numbers derived from experiments on mice lead to assessments of 1–15 days' loss of human life per rem received. On this basis, up to 8 years of life would be lost by an occupational worker receiving the maximum permissible dose of 200 rems in a lifetime. Neary (4) argues that the absolute value in mice and men might well be the same, namely 0.08 days per rem, and this unlike the former estimate is compatible with the facts as observed.

Malignant Change

Practically no tissue in the body is exempt from malignant transformation or cancer, but spontaneous cancer is commoner in certain sites than others. Possibly some day we will uncover the fundamental difference between the normal and malignant cell, that is we will discover the cause of cancer, that unique phenomenon, if it exists. In the meanwhile we must recognize that just as there is a wide variety of tissues within the body, each with many recognizably different types of malignant transformation, there are likely to be scores of causes of cancer or accessories to the crime. Most of cancer research of the past few decades has been investigation into the natural history of cancers and the role of influences, originating from without and within the body, on the induction or progression of the processes. We thus speak of carcinogenic agents, meaning physical, chemical, and even biological entities which under the right circumstances can effect the malignant transformation.

The most well-known agents are chemical, notably coal tar derivatives. Following the observation of the last century that chimney sweeps were subject to cancer of the skin, a search for carcinogenic agents in soot was logical and ultimately successful. The active agents isolated from soot and their chemical analogues will, when painted on the skin of experimental animals, ultimately give rise in a high proportion of cases to cancer at the site of the painting. If they are injected into the blood stream, they do not reproduce the occupational disease. Instead they give rise to an increased incidence of "leukemia." There is good reason therefore to believe that substances like benzpyrene are general carcinogens and an action by them on bronchial mucous membrane is invoked to explain the statistical correlation between cancer of the "lung" and cigarette smoking.

Physical agents, particularly ionizing radiation, can be similarly more or less universally carcinogenic. Localized irradiation from without or that derived from radioactive materials deposited within tissues has been recorded as producing cancer in dozens of sites. However, when the irradiation is generalized over the whole body, certain sites of election of subsequent development of cancer become manifest. Doubtless, internal factors then begin to influence the process, as presumably they do also in the spontaneous cancers. Among these internal factors must be listed the hormonal secretions of the ductless glands—pituitary, thyroid, adrenal, sex glands, and thymus—which influence the cellular activity of each other and of diverse tissues in the body at large.

There is a strong body of opinion among pathologists which incriminates—as accessory factors to cancerous change—cycles of cellular activity, with bouts of overactivity alternating with involution or destruction. These may be physiological, like the changes in breast tissue under the influence of sex hormones, or pathological, like the gastric cancer complicating simple peptic ulceration, or a complex of the two, such as cancer of the uterine neck in parous women—physiological cycles associated with lacerations and recurrent bacterial infections. In the ulcerative conditions bacteria and their toxins may play a role, probably secondary, in carcinogenesis. But a primary role for viruses is well-established, if not for man certainly in the animal kingdom. The role of viruses in the causation of fowl leukemia (39) has been accepted for 50 years. For almost as long the Rous (40) agent has been known to induce a rapidly growing, solid, malignant sarcoma in fowls. The phenomenon was shown not to be confined to birds: simple tumors of mammals were transmitted by cell-free solutions. Twenty-five years ago Bittner (41) showed the association of viruses with mammalian tumors was not confined to simple growths. He demonstrated that cancers of the breast in certain strains of laboratory mice were associated with an agent transmitted by maternal milk to suckling offspring. Ten years ago Gross (42) began marshaling the evidence for a viral causation of mouse leukemia, though for a long time his was a voice crying in the wilderness. His thesis is now generally accepted. The virus is considered as transmitted to offspring via the egg. Since these strains of mice continue to survive, the developmental period is long. In the last few years a lot more tumor-producing viruses have been found, perhaps the most intriguing being the so-called polyoma (43) viruses, as injection of them into newborn animals produces in a very short time a wide variety of malignant tumors in different individual hosts. However, as far as I am aware, in spite of a number of suggestive circumstances, there are as yet no accredited association of viruses with malignant tumors in man.

LEUKEMIA

Since it is patent that all malignant conditions cannot be discussed in this presentation, I propose to concentrate on "leukemia." This is far from being a typical malignancy: in fact not so long ago there were sizable bodies of opinion against its classification as a malignant disease. It is not a single entity, clinically, pathologically, or in comparative anatomy. But it is a fashionable condition for study at the present time because considerable advances in our understanding of it are being made; moreover, in Western civilizations its incidence has been increasing, and there is an association between leukemia and ionizing radiation.

It is difficult enough to define a cancer. I was taught that it was an "autonomous new growth" that is, in terms of behavior, selfish, serving its own ends and not those of the integrated organism as a whole, and not subject to the normal discipline of the body. In general the constituent cells of a cancer tend to be immature and undifferentiated for special function, invasive of their surroundings, often metastasizing, that is colonizing at a distance when constituent cells are carried from the site of origin by blood, lymph, or the surgeon's knife, and in the case of experimental animals transmissible from one to another by implantation. None of these features is by itself diagnostic. The composite picture leads the pathologist to his opinion, and the specialist's opinion, while usually right, may be wrong.

"Leukemia" is similar or, to coin a phrase, more so. It is a malignant transformation of the blood-forming tissues, which normally are the bone marrow in the human adult and the lymphoid masses. In the embryo, however, the liver and splenic pulp are also hemopoietic; this state persists in some animals, as does the potentiality in man. In the clinically developed state of leukemia, the whole or a large part of the marrow-like (myeloid) tissues are involved in myeloid leukemia and the whole or a large part of the lymphoid tissues in lymphatic leukemia. It is not certain whether the processes start in a single focus and spread or whether there is a multicentric origin. However, one of the recent developments is in knowledge of the physiological recirculation of blood cells and blood-forming cells.

Red blood corpuscles, which are not true cells as they have lost their nuclei, are formed in the bone marrow and pushed into the circulation where they perform their job of carrying oxygen. Normally they stay in circulation and persist for a fixed period of about 4 months, when they are replaced.

Granular white cells are also formed in the marrow. They belong to the mobile antibacterial defenses of the body; they can creep out of the circulation and are apparently lost from the circulation in a statistically random fashion.

Lymphocytes, non-granular white cells, are formed in lymphoid tissue and enter the blood stream. They too are mobile and can wander out into tissue; but it appears that they can return to lymphoid tissue, which is widely dispersed in the body, perhaps for rest and refreshment, and then recirculate.

Monocytes, a minority population of non-granular white cells, are scavengers of debris. They are formed in the marrow and possibly elsewhere too.

There was a time, not very long ago, when it was generally taught that only the mature cells escaped from the production sites to appear in the blood and that the presence of primitive cells there indicated enormous overactivity, perhaps reactive to some severe stress on the respective blood-forming tissue, perhaps malignant or "leukemic."

Thus leukemia was a malignant transformation of some hemopoietic tissue with a spill-over of primitive cells into the blood which presumably could metastasize almost anywhere (1 [1961]).

The *British Medical Journal* in a leading article recently summarized the situation for M.D.'s.

Three years ago C. E. Ford and his colleagues [44*] following up the clue provided by observations on leukaemic mice [45], observed changes in the chromosomes in one human case of acute leukaemia. The cytological abnormality was detected in a culture of bone-marrow. In the *Journal* this week (. . . .) Dr. A. G. Baikie and his colleagues [46] have reviewed their observations on a series of 31 cases, from 22 of which satisfactory preparations were available. Not all cases of leukaemia provide myeloid material suitable for analysis, though a notable technical advance has been the discovery that cells which can be induced to undergo mitotic division are obtainable from peripheral blood of both normal and leukaemia subjects [47]. Thus Baikie and colleagues examined preparations

---

* The numbering of references in this excerpt has been changed from the original in order to agree with the numeration of references in the present volume.

from both peripheral blood and marrow. As a rule, it can be said that the two sources give the same qualitative picture.

At present, interpretation of the cells seen in the peripheral blood is still somewhat obscure. The presence of "blast" cells in the circulating blood has long been one of the criteria of diagnosis of leukaemia. They have been recognized from finding atypical cells which on morphological grounds are called myeloblasts, lymphoblasts, primitive monocytes, or stem cells. It is rare to find one spontaneously in mitosis. Now, however, it is recognized that even in normal subjects some of the typical circulating leucocytes with the appearance of monocytes or large lymphocytes are primitive in the sense that they are actively synthesizing D.N.A. [48]. These presumably are the cells which can be induced in culture to divide and show their normal set of chromosomes to contrast with the leukaemic cells, which may have chromosomes abnormal in number, form, or both.

The old concept was that the leukaemic cells were a spill-over or metastasis from the malignant myeloid tissue. Are the cells which are normally synthesizing D.N.A. a similar and physiological metastasis? And if so what is their function? J. F. Loutit, [49] taking as a model certain biochemical cycles (like the Krebs cycle), postulated that a similar cellular cycle occurs in haemopoiesis. In the marrow multipotent stem cells provide a lymphopoietic line of cells as well as the conventional erythropoietic and granulopoietic lines—this is the standard monophyletic hypothesis. The primitive lymphoid cells are carried by the blood stream to lymph tissue, where they mature, re-enter the blood, and ultimately reach the marrow to expire and return D.N.A. or other essential material to the factory. This hypothesis was based on experiments with mice in which the myeloid and lymphoid tissues were made aplastic with X-rays and then restored with intravascular injections of active myeloid tissue from a donor.

But it is now seen to be incomplete, for R. A. Popp [50] has shown that a sufficiently large dose of leucocytes from normal peripheral blood will also restore erythropoiesis. Presumably, therefore, the primitive D.N.A.-synthesizing cells in the peripheral blood are not limited to lymphopoietic cells but include erythropoietic and granulopoietic (or stem) cells also. This accords with the fact that their morphology has been reported as mixed—monocytic or large lymphocytic.

While an export of lymphopoietic cells from the marrow is explicable as a sole or supplementary means of producing lymphocytes, what is the explanation of an export of myeloid cells? Or is it an import of primitive stem cells from some dispersed mesoblastic tissue supplementing the marrow? On the model of L. G. Lajtha and R. Oliver [51], limited by them to the erythron but applicable to other myeloid cell lines, such supplementation would seem unnecessary. Moreover, D. W. H. Barnes and colleagues [52] have shown with irradiated mice that a total of a few million myeloid cells (presumably containing only a few tens of thousands of stem cells) on serial passage is for some years the sole source of the myeloid and lymphoid tissue. The weight of evidence therefore suggests that the normal primitive cells are an export from the marrow, and the same seems to apply to leukaemia. In the cases discussed by Baikie and colleagues, though atypical cells were found in the circulation, tissue-cultures of skin, presumably of primitive mesoblastic cells, showed normal chromosomal patterns.

It seems therefore that the extrusion of primitive cells from the site of production into the peripheral blood is not a specific phenomenon of leukaemia. Indeed, it is well known that many leukaemias are aleukaemic. The characteristic of the disease lies in the production of abnormal cells. How the relatively constant chromosomal abnormality in chronic myeloid leukaemia [53] and the variable abnormality seen with the light microscope in acute leukaemia are related to the fundamental causes still remains to be elucidated.

Thus the presence of primitive cells in the peripheral blood, in small numbers it is true, is not pathognomonic of leukemia, and some true "leukemias" do not manifest the spill-over of primitive cells into the blood. The diagnosis of leukemia is becoming a matter of much more sophistication than formerly.

Once it was sufficient in the frankly leukemic cases to categorize by time and cell-type. Acute leukemias were expected to run a rapid course of weeks or at most months and were stigmatized by very primitive cells in the peripheral blood. Cases of chronic leukemia might live for years, and their abnormal cells in the blood, though often very numerous, were intermediate in maturity. The cell-types were determined from their form or staining as myeloid (in the sense of granular-leucocyte-forming), lymphatic, mono-cytic, and even, tautologically, erythroleukemic.

Now it involves study of the marrow by needle puncture and perhaps biopsy of lymphoid or other tissues. Moreover, as the *British Medical Journal's* leading article infers, it now presumes a look at microanatomy of the cells, the chromosomes. The ability to visualize the chromosomes stems largely from the work of my colleague Ford following the need to do so for laboratory studies in mouse-radiation genetics (Carter *et al.* [54]). Irradiation of testes had resulted in sperm which on fertilization of normal eggs had led to offspring with abnormal associations of genes; that is the irradiation of sperm-producing cells had led to chromosome-breaks which healed by cross union or translocation. The need, therefore, was to confirm the association found by breeding tests with direct cytological observation. Ford was able to do this in one case. If chromosomes could thus be visualized in spermatogonia, they could also be visualized in hemopoietic tissue, and the radiation-induced visible translocated chromosome because useful as a cell-population marker (55). We were able to show that myeloid tissue from these mice could on intravenous injection recolonize not only the bone marrow but lymphoid tissues of mice where these tissues had been depopulated by large doses of X-rays, normally lethal. We now have experience of mice like these, with blood-forming tissues formed of cells with a visibly atypical chromosome (see Fig. 8). They are not more liable to develop leukemia than mice restored with normal marrow.

Breakage of a chromosome and reunion are thus in themselves not sufficient to induce leukemia even in the cellular environment of an irradiated mouse. Nevertheless when the cells of the abnormal tissues of mice affected with leukemia, spontaneous or radiation-induced, were examined cytologically, abnormalities of the chromosome complement were identifiable in the majority (45) (see Fig. 11). Thus leukemia of the mouse apparently results in chromosomal abnormalities of which many must be translocations; or, if the translocations be related to cause rather than effect, one particular chromosome or part of it must be involved. There is no evidence of this as yet from work on the mouse, which, as far as identification of chromosomes is concerned, is not a particularly favorable animal to work with, as most of the chromosomes are very much alike in form.

When we return to man, however, we have a more readily analyzable situation with regard to the chromosomes. Tjio and Levan (56) and Ford and Hamerton (57), both in 1956, were able for the first time to get satisfactory preparations of human cells allowing them to enumerate the chromosomes as 46 (hitherto 48 was the number favored) and to identify the normal array or karyotype. This has now been systematized by international agreement in the "Denver classification" (58) (see Figs. 1 and 2). The array of chromosomes is remarkably constant from cell to cell in the normal subject, though a small proportion of cells in any preparation may have some deficiency of chromosomes due to artifacts in making the preparation. It might be expected that the proportion of really abnormal arrays would increase with age of the subject, and a preliminary indication of this has been seen by Court Brown (59).

While the normal individual has a normal array, it is now evident that certain abnormal individuals have a congenitally abnormal array. These usually characterize clinical syndromes of abnormal development. Bulking large among these are disturbances of development of the sex organs. The normal female is characterized by two X chromosomes and the male by an XY constitution. But individuals with constitution XXY (Klinefelter's syndrome—47 chromosomes) and XO (Turner's syndrome—45 chromosomes) are now commonly recognized, and the series is being extended—XXX, XXXY, etc. The basic cause is reckoned to be failure of the chromosomes to find their way—non-disjunction—to the right pole during one of the cell divisions in the production of the germ cell (see chap. i and Fig. 7). A similar fault can occur in early embryonic life resulting in a so-called mosaic individual, e.g. XO.XX.

Another group tends to be characterized by multiple abnormalities of development, including those of the nervous system. Prominent among them and the earliest to be identified with abnormal chromosomal constitution was Mongolism. In this condition there are again 47 chromosomes per cell, with triplication of chromosome 21. For our purpose it is important to note that it has been recognized for some years that Mongols are more prone than normal subjects to develop leukemia (see Fig. 6).

Given that methods had been developed for analyzing the numbers and some of the morphological features of human chromosomes, it was obvious that the patterns of human leukemic cells would be investigated. Ford, Jacobs, and Lajtha (44) made the first essay followed closely by groups in the U.S.A. In the United Kingdom Jacobs followed up the initial study at Harwell using the much more extensive human material available in a unit with clinical attachments under Dr. Court Brown in Edinburgh. These studies have confirmed that, as in mice, so in men leukemic cells may have chromosomal abnormalities (see Fig. 5).

In acute leukemia of apparently variable cell-type, structural faults may be seen. They seem, like those in murine leukemia, to be inconstant from case to case and presumably specific for that case, certainly at the relevant time. In general they are suggestive of some rather late effect, secondary to the disease. Most cases of leukemia in Mongols are of this acute type, and, while the specific triplication of chromosome 21 is present, there is nothing specific as far as the leukemia is concerned.

On the other hand, from Philadelphia (60) came the initial report to be confirmed from Edinburgh (53) that in cases of chronic myeloid leukemia an apparently specific defect of a small chromosome, which could be number 21, was evident (see Fig. 10). This has caused some speculation about the relation of this chromosome to granulocytes. It is still speculation.

The general situation today concerning chromosomes in relation to malignancy is one of flux. Knowledge advances by fits and starts. It is not fundamentally a new observation that malignancy of cells is associated with abnormalities of mitosis and of chromosomes. Awareness of this goes back half a century. What is new is the now greatly improved techniques that allow dogmatism on the regularity of normal cells, with which the irregularity of malignant cells can be contrasted, and that permit characterization of the specific details of the abnormalities of chromosomes according to the individual tumor.

An abnormal chromosome number or the presence of an abnormal chromosome betokens an abnormal array of constituent genes.

This may involve an excess or deficiency of normal genes; it may include alteration, that is mutation of genes; it certainly means a change in balance of genes compared with the normal cell.

Abnormalities of mitosis of some types can provide the means whereby this unbalance arises.

The reawakened interest in mitotic and chromosomal abnormalities stems from experimental work in the laboratory. The immediate factor in the case of leukemia was study of the detail of cells from leukemic mice. It is therefore appropriate at this stage to review murine leukemia to recapitulate some things which have already been noted and to compare and contrast it with human leukemia. Study of the mouse or other experimental animal may provide further clues for future clinical research.

COMPARISON WITH MURINE LEUKEMIA

First we should note that the term *leukemia* in the mouse is often used in what used to be called a loose sense, that is the frank presence of atypical cells in the circulating blood is not so characteristic as in human leukemia. But we have noted that more and more cases of human leukemia are being diagnosed even though aleukemic. The florid case of human leukemia may have a leucocyte count 10 to 100 times greater than the average normal, and of these cells too many, anything up to 100 per cent, can be primitive and abnormal. But nowadays an increasingly large percentage of cases are recognized that never manifest this state. In the mouse the florid leukemic state is a rarity, but it is not uncommon, particularly in the terminal stages, for the leucocyte count to be raised several fold above the average normal, and for 10 per cent or so of the cells to be atypical.

The greatest numbers of human leukemia are of the myeloid or lymphoid type; only a minority is classified as monocytic or erythroleukemic. In the laboratory strains of mice only lymphoid and myeloid types are generally recognized, and of these the lymphoid is greatly preponderant.

The diseases tend to affect mice in the middle to the end of the normal life spans of mouse colonies. Among the lymphoid, one type, which is commonly called the lymphoblastic, has a maximum incidence in susceptible strains around 1 year of age. It may manifest itself purely as a localized tumor of the thymus or as such a tumor with a more or less generalized dissemination in the lymphoid and myeloid tissues or as the generalized state without special localization in the thymus. Another type, reticulosarcoma, affects elderly mice, is often confined to the abdominal regions of the lymphatic tissues, and may have a protracted course. Because the features of both lymphoblastic and reticular cell-types are mainly tumefacient rather than leukemic, the conditions may be more accurately described as lymphomas than leukemias; but the distribution of the malignant cells, particularly in the lymphoblastic types, in reticuloendothelial tissues as seen under the microscope is so similar to what is found in human leukemia that one judges that the underlying mechanisms ought to be very similar.

In the types where the thymus is involved, it has become patent that the thymus plays a very important role. This type of leukemia is common in many laboratory strains. In the past, for investigational purposes, selection for leukemia was practiced so that abundant material would be available for research. Two commonly used strains, known as AK and C58, have been developed and are now maintained by strict inbreeding; in them the death rate from this form of leukemia is around 90 per cent. It was from AK mice that Gross obtained the cell-free extract, which was able to induce this leukemia in other strains with a low natural incidence, and so developed the virus theory of the causation of this type of leukemia.

If AK mice have their thymuses removed surgically while young, they no longer develop this leukemia in later life. The thymus is a lymphoid organ which regresses naturally with age. This process is not so rapid in the mouse as in man, where it used to be reckoned that it was atrophic by puberty. Recently there has been some reassessment of this dogma from data obtained at autopsy on young men, battle casualties, and regression in man may not be so complete or as rapid as once taught. The maximum development of the thymus occurs in the infant and young animal. Fifty years ago the large size of this gland in young children dying unexpectedly led to concept of a disease—*status thymolymphaticus*. The hypothesis was exploded more than a generation ago, but until recently earnest physicians have been looking for enlarged thymuses in infants and children so that they could have them blasted with X-rays. This has been incriminated in Chicago and Rochester as a cause of post-irradiation malignancy in these children at older ages.

Since nobody is certain what is the function of the thymus, ablation is a very reasonable operation on the experimental animal in an attempt to find out what is the result of deficiency of the gland. It is odd but real that its excision in the AK mice should be beneficial in preventing the expected development of a leukemic state presumably induced by virus passaged from mother to her offspring. It is generally accepted too that the thymus produces thymocytes, which are undistinguishable from ordinary lymphocytes in appearance, but which may be functionally different; the thymus certainly seems to have a lower immunological capacity than other lymphoid tissue. Removing its lymphocytopoietic activity is unlikely to be noticeable, as the body has enormous reserves of lymphoid tissue. Sir Howard Florey (61) discovered this experimentally many years ago by attempts to remove surgically all lymphoid tissue. Metcalf (62), another Australian, attributes to the thymus the secretion of a lymphopoietic stimulating factor into the blood stream, but though his experiments are convincing this factor must be a refinement not an essential, as the thymus is dispensable; perhaps it is even an embarrassment, for it is found in excess in AK mice.*

It seems, therefore, that the exogenous virus and endogenous thymus collaborate in the production of the "thymic" type of

* J. F. A. P. Miller (*Lancet*, **2**: 748. 1961), another Australian, has now shown that extirpation of the mouse's thymus at birth leads to failure of development of the other lymphoid tissues with consequent immunological upset. This technical masterpiece identifies the role of the thymus as the initial organizer of the lymphoid system: its work done, it can atrophy in adolescence.

natural leukemia. It has been noted that radiation has a leukemogenic effect on all strains of mice and that there are optimal
schedules of irradiation for the induction—usually a series of doses
of moderate sizes given at intervals. My colleague Mole (34) has
made the interesting observation that a further large dose of
X-rays at the end of the optimal course will prevent the expected
development of leukemia. One way of explaining this would be to
say that the optimal course of radiation has transformed a considerable number of cells so that any of them can act as the focus for
future leukemia; the large dose of radiation then kills most of the
transformed cells. This explanation is, however, probably too
facile.

The administration of the optimal leukemogenic course of irradiation to thymectomized mice also fails to produce the expected
leukemia, so that the thymus has a collaboratory function in this
type of leukemia too. As Kaplan and his colleagues (63) have
shown, this function can be restored to the thymectomized mice
after the course of irradiation by implantation under the skin of a
normal thymus gland. To insure survival of the grafted gland, one
must choose it from a donor that is immunologically compatible,
for example from an animal of the same inbred strain. In fact
Kaplan used as the thymectomized irradiated host a hybrid of 2
pure strains (C57BL × C3H) and as donated thymus that from
the parental type C57BL. He was able to show that subsequent
leukemias were of the C57BL antigenic type. Others including
ourselves (64, 65) have shown that this is not invariably so, that
about half are of host type, half of donor type, but the principle
remains firm—the leukemia can arise in these circumstances from
cells which have not been irradiated. In other words environmental
factors in the irradiated host are of considerable importance.

Does virus play a role with the thymus in the elicitation of
radiation-induced leukemia of the mouse? Gross obtained his virus
originally from a leukemic AK mouse. Although we (65) were
unable to demonstrate by Gross' technique a virus in our radiation-
induced leukemic mice, Gross (66) himself, certainly more experi-

enced in this practice than ourselves, has done so on occasion with his C3H mice made leukemic by irradiation, and Kaplan (67) had similarly had some successes with C57BL mice.*

The test for the virus is at present a biological assay. The cell-free extract is injected into susceptible mice. Newborn mice are the most susceptible recipients, and a positive test consists in the development of a statistically significant excess of leukemias in the injected mice compared with controls. Mature mice will normally not show this phenomenon, presumably because the virus is not sufficiently numerous or sufficiently avid. By repeated passage of the virus through susceptible hosts, Gross (68) has been able to increase the potency of cell-free extracts obtained so that even mature mice as recipients will give positive results. Thus, in general, a test of this sort, if positive, can be taken as evidence in favor of the presence of virus in the extract under review, and, if negative, does not exclude the presence of virus.

Virus particles if reasonably abundant can be identified by means of the electron microscope. Once again, however, failure to identify virus does not exclude its presence. We thus have apparent thresholds above which a positive reading is accepted. But, as with thresholds for radiation-effect discussed earlier, we are logically in a difficult position when we consider subthreshold levels. Is there ever an absolute zero and is the biological response at levels between zero and some apparent threshold entirely comparable with that above the threshold?

My instinctive feeling on this question of virus would be that from time to time in individual mice there may well be an absolute absence of this particular virus. In the ordinary laboratory, housing multiple stocks, however, the virus is almost certainly present and under the usual conditions of maintenance there will be occasions for transfer. Most individuals of most stocks will be able to resist by natural or acquired immunity the multiplication of the

---

* A. J. Dalton, L. W. Law, J. B. Moloney, and R. A. Manaker (*J. Nat. Cancer Inst.*, 27: 747. 1961) in an electron-microscopic study have found vuris particles in tissues of AKR mice with spontaneous leukemia, in mice with virus-induced leukemias of several types, but not in radition-induced leukemia of C57BL mice.

virus to biologically effective levels. The AK and other stocks of this kind must have, genetically determined, some defect in their mechanisms of resistance. Their resistance cannot be nil or they would not live to their average age of a year or thereabouts: it must decline with age.

Individuals who can react by classical acquired immunity can probably quickly build up an effective and permanent resistance, just as man can to, say, virus of yellow fever. Burnet (69), whose opinions must carry great weight in matters of immunology, argues cogently that under these circumstances in man virus is no longer present and that the permanent immunity is due to the presence of clones of lymphoid cells activated by the infection. But the proof of absolute absence of virus is lacking and, because of the difficulty of demonstrating zero, may never be attained. We are well aware, on the other hand, in bacterial diseases of the existence of "carriers." The infection has occurred, with or without overt manifestation of the disease; the organism is destroyed by the acquired immunological processes in loci where they can act, but the organism persists in pockets, e.g. the gall bladder of typhoid carriers. Privileged sites such as these are well recognized by immunologists. Are there no pockets for viruses, from which a leak into the system would continue to activate the specific clones of lymphoid cells to maintain an effective level of general corporeal immunity but into which the clonal cells or their soluble products cannot reversely penetrate? For the maintenance of immunological tolerance to foreign antigen, which might be considered the obverse of immunity, there is now good evidence that the continued presence of antigen is necessary.

I have formerly postulated, as have others, that the mice like the AK strain may be immunologically tolerant of the virus. Gross (70) has argued for the vertical transmission of virus from mother to offspring via the egg, and this could have initiated tolerance; but under these circumstances we might expect the virus to multiply explosively with early manifestation of leukemia, as occurs when serially passaged virus is given to susceptible recipients. Vertical transmission may well occur, but it does not seem to me

to be an essential. Provided there is occasion for repeated exposure
to the virus, it is acceptable in the hypothesis of clonal selection
that any acquired immunity that is built up, allowing the mouse
to survive for many months, can be exhausted and that clones
poorly reacting or unreactive be selected. An explanation in these
terms might account for the observation that C3H mice frequently
injected with, or surgically joined by the operation of parabiosis to,
hybrid (C3H × A)F₁ mice may later accept skin grafts from
C3H × A donor (71). It should however be noted that this is still
the exception and not the rule.

Getting away from speculation I should think it fairly firm that,
if virus is an essential factor in natural murine leukemia, immunity
natural and acquired is involved. Irradiation is known to affect
particularly those reticuloendothelial tissues that are concerned
with immunity. A substantial dose of radiation will lead to a permanent weakening of immunological response. This may not be
demonstrable in the case of strong antigens which produce a
vigorous response but can be against weak antigens. Perhaps virus
is a weak antigen for all mice, especially the naturally susceptible
like AK.

However, whether or not virus is an essential factor in the
radiation-induced thymic type of leukemia, the role of the thymus
seems similar to that in spontaneous leukemia, in that thymectomy
abolishes the development of leukemia. Kaplan (72) many years
ago, reviewing the role of the thymus, argued that disorderly recovery of the thymus following regression due to leukemogenic
agents (exogenous chemicals, hormones, X-rays, etc.) was a factor
in the subsequent evolution of the leukemia. In radiobiological
studies the leukemia occurs following irradiation of the whole body
but not following the same exposure with the sole exception of
some shielded bone marrow. Thus Kaplan postulated that a bone-
marrow factor is essential for orderly recovery of the thymus. My
(73) emendation was that the bone-marrow factor was in all probability comparable with that required in other radiobiological
experiments for recovery of the mouse itself following lethal irradi-

ation, not humoral but a phenomenon of cellular reseeding. Current work by my colleagues (74, 75) indicates that the lethally irradiated mouse that is given as restorative therapy a mixture of myeloid and lymphoid cells will in the early stages of recovery restitute its thymus from the myeloid cells but the rest of its lymphoid tissue from the lymphoid cells. Fichtelius (76) provides evidence that thymic cells pass to the splenic pulp, perhaps to become immunologically active. The suggestion is, therefore, that the thymus is an intermediate in a cellular cycle from bone marrow to immune mechanism. It may not be essential to life but could be a booster for the young and vulnerable because of immunological inexperience.

From the foregoing, which naturally enough is not the whole story but merely the bits which have most impressed me, the general conclusion must be that, though virus and thymus have to be fitted into the composite picture of radiation induced lymphoid leukemia in the mouse, we cannot yet see the picture as a whole but only pieces of a jigsaw puzzle.

As noted above, not all radiation-induced lymphoid leukemia primarily involves the thymus. From my own laboratory Mole (77) has identified that mice about 2 months old at the beginning of a leukemogenic course of irradiation die with "thymic" leukemia around 9 months, more or less, later. Other leukemias tend to be spread more evenly, with deaths between 3 and 30 months later. Thymic leukemia with Mole's radiation-schedule was induced only above a threshold of 500 r; generalized leukemias occurred in those mice receiving less than 500 r.

Specifying doses only in terms of the integral amount received— e.g., 500 r as above—is valid when the schedules of irradiation are comparable. It may not always be so. In a formal experiment to test this, Mole (78) gave different groups of mice an integrated total of 1,000 r of X-rays over a period of 4 weeks. But the dose-rate—and therefore the radiation-free time between fractions— was varied from 81 r/hour intermittently to 1.3 r/hour continuously. The incidence of leukemia varied from 40 per cent (within

15 months of the start of irradiation) in the first group to 5 per cent in the last compared with 2 per cent incidence in unirradiated controls.

"Myeloid" leukemia is very much less commonly seen naturally or induced by radiation. As with the "lymphoid" type it tends to be found in certain strains, for example RF. Upton and the group at Oak Ridge (79) have reported on induction of both myeloid and lymphoid leukemia in this strain. The following is their summary:

1. The susceptibility of mice of the RF strain to radiation-induced myeloid leukemia and lymphomas was studied under a variety of experimental conditions.

2. Although the rate of induction of both diseases varied in relation to the dose of radiation, the relation between disease incidence and dose was not the same for both neoplasms; neither was it linear over the dosage range 0–500 r.

3. On fractionation of a given dose of radiation, the rate of induction of leukemia varied depending on the total dose, dose per exposure, interval between exposures, and hematologic type of leukemia produced.

4. Shielding of the pelvis and lower extremities during irradiation of the remainder of the body greatly inhibited the induction of myeloid leukemia as well as lymphomas.

5. Susceptibility to lymphoma induction, which is higher in females than in males, was decreased by ovariectomy but was not affected by orchidectomy. Susceptibility to the induction of myeloid leukemia, which is higher in males than in females, was not significantly affected by gonadectomy in either sex. The sex differences in the susceptibility to induction of lymphomas and myeloid leukemia persisted even after removal of the gonads.

6. Removal of the spleen before irradiation greatly lowered susceptibility to the induction of myeloid leukemia but did not influence the induction of lymphomas.

7. Newborn mice were resistant to the induction of myeloid leukemia despite susceptibility to lymphoma formation, whereas the reverse was true of mice irradiated at 6 months of age.

8. Removal of the thymus before irradiation, which eliminated the induction of thymic lymphomas, permitted the induction of lymphomas in extra thymic lymphoid tissues but did not influence the formation of myeloid leukemia.

Though the thymus might not be involved as in the lymphoblastic leukemia, virus has been incriminated. While Gross was exploring cell-free extracts from leukemic tissue of the AK mouse, Graffi (80) in Berlin was making extracts from some long-established and passaged mouse tumors, sarcoma I and II (Landschütz). From this source he obtained an extract which induced leukemia in his test strain. This leukemia is apparently an acute myeloid variety and gives chloromatous deposits reminiscent of some human acute leukemias.

HUMAN LEUKEMIA—INCIDENCE

Leukemia has been diagnosed at all ages in man.

Infants.—There are now quite a considerable number of individual case reports of infants having been born with leukemia from apparently healthy mothers. I am not aware, however, of any collection of these data for an assessment of the rate of incidence of such congenital leukemia.

Children.—In childhood, leukemia is not uncommon and is receiving increasing attention. It is the commonest malignant condition in children and clinically is almost always of the rapidly progressive acute type. It may be listed as myeloid or lymphoid or unspecified, but it is doubtful how valid the available figures are since the classification of the predominant cell depends very much on the opinions held by the diagnosing clinician or pathologist. There would, however, be general agreement that, just as the clinical course is rapid, so the degree of differentiation of the predominant cell, which is the indicator of the definitive type, is minimal. In many cases the predominant cell is small and may mimic the normal small lymphocyte, but in reality the cell is probably an undifferentiated primitive cell not peculiar to, but more commonly found, in children.

It has been pointed out that the diagnosis of leukemia is dependent on sophistication. The mortality of infants has always been high, and until recently mortality in childhood was also high from acute infections. Many of the deaths may in fact have been due to leukemia but certified as from one of the much more common acute illnesses of childhood. With the increasing availability of pathological services in countries with a high degree of civilization, it is to be expected that leukemia would be more readily diagnosable than in those countries with less adequate medical facilities or than in the same country in the past. For example in England, Wood (81) describes graphically the improvements that have occurred in a rural area since 1948, and the consequent difficulty of interpretation of recorded incidence of leukemia as obtained in recent surveys. One might conclude that apparent increases in the rate of leukemia might not be real, but that declining rates and perhaps even steady rates indicate a real decline. In this limited area of Cornwall, Wood finds no increase in leukemia in children in the recent 12-year period.

However, in surveys covering much larger areas and therefore much more diverse environments, there seems to be fairly general agreement of an increase in diagnosed leukemia in children in the last 30 years (see Table 1). Stewart and her colleagues (82) in

TABLE 1*

DEATH RATES FROM LEUKEMIA IN ENGLAND AND WALES, 1931–35 TO 1955–59, BY AGE

AGE (YEARS)	DEATH RATE PER 1,000,000 PERSONS†			
	1931–35	1945–49	1950–54	1955–59
0–4	24	41	46	43
5–9	16	24	30	33
10–14	13	19	21	22
15–19	13	20	22	21
20–24	11	15	18	19
25–29	12	14	18	21
30–34	13	20	18	21
35–39	12	21	25	27
40–44	18	25	32	34
45–49	23	35	38	40
50–54	27	41	47	50
55–59	35	53	70	74
60–64	41	74	94	106
65–69	52	85	128	136
70–74	43	88	137	184
75–79	34	82	149	223
80 and over	20	49	115	210

* Reproduced with permission from Court Brown, W. M. and Doll, R. (92).
† Standardized for a population of equal numbers of men and women.

England and others elsewhere have given considerable attention to this. Stewart *et al.* summarize their first survey, in which an attempt was made to trace all children in England and Wales who had died of leukemia or cancer before their tenth birthday during the years 1953–55, as follows:

The pre-natal and post-natal experiences of a large group of children who recently died of malignant diseases have been compared, point by point, with the experiences of a similar group of live children.

The frequency of three pre-natal events—namely, direct foetal irradiation, virus infections and threatened abortion—was significantly higher among the dead children than among the live children.

One other pre-natal influence—namely, excessive maternal age—appears to increase the risk of leukaemia in childhood and to be related to the fact that this disease and mongolism tend to occur together.

The frequency of three post-natal events—namely, X-ray exposures in infancy, acute pulmonary infections and severe injuries—was significantly higher for children who subsequently died of leukaemia than for other children. In the "pre-antibiotic era" some of these children might have died before showing signs of the leukaemia.

The health of the mothers and the home background of the children were not significantly different in the two groups, but there were minor points of difference in the family histories of cancer and leukaemia.

Our final conclusions are that foetal irradiation does not account for the recent increase in childhood malignancies, but the finding of a case excess for this event does underline the need to use minimum doses for essential medical X-ray examinations and treatments.

Since we are interested in the relationship of ionizing radiation to the induction of leukemia, it is worth noting the actual words used by these authors as they are often quoted as implying a greater role to radiation than in fact they did. In another place they say:

On this showing children who have been X-rayed *in utero* are . . . twice as likely to die of a malignant disease before their tenth birthday as other children. Since at the present time about one in every 1200 children in Britain die in this way, it follows that less than one in a thousand of the pre-natal X-ray examinations performed in recent years have led to death from malignant disease before the age of 10 years.

Stewart (83) has continued to examine the statistical evidence. She notes that the peak of the death rate for leukemia is early in childhood (ages 3–4), like that of retinoblastomas and renal tumors (Fig. 21). She also notes that, while the recorded death rate of leukemia in childhood has risen in the last generation, that from pneumonia has declined in a reciprocal fashion (Fig. 22). These data are in accord with her present working hypothesis:

1. Malignant diseases are initiated by X-rays and other mutagens before conception (prezygotic), during pregnancy (prenatal), or after birth (post-natal). The last two groups correspond to post-zygotic cancers and leukaemias.

2. In childhood the chief promoter of malignant diseases is the cell

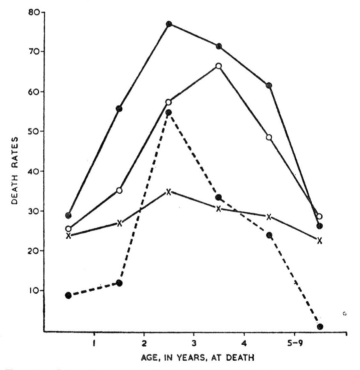

Fig. 21.—Mortality rates. Leukemias, retinoblastomas, and renal tumors. O————O , Leukemias (1950–57), rate per million, E. and W. (England and Wales) X————X, Leukemias (1930–39), rate per million, E. and W. ●------● , Eye tumors (1950–57), rate per 10 million, U.S.A. ●————● , Renal tumors (1950–57), rate per million, E. and W. (From A. Stewart, in *Brit. Med. J.*, 1 [1961]: 452, Fig. 1.)

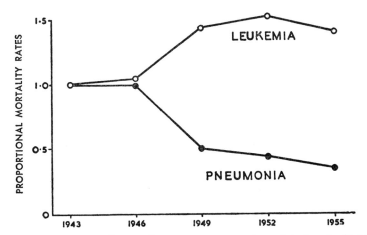

Fɪɢ. 22.—Proportional mortality rates: pneumonia and leukemia (0–10 years). (From A. Stewart, in *Brit. Med. J.*, 1 [1961]: 452, Fig. 4.)

stress of embryogenesis. Consequently most childhood cancers and leukaemias are prezygotic.

3. At all ages the leucocyte stress provoked by infections is a promoter of leukaemias. By increasing susceptibility to infections mongolism acts as an indirect promoter of leukaemias. Because mongolism is an inherited condition (Lejeune, Gautier, and Turpin [84*], 1959) it has more opportunity to affect prezygotic than post-zygotic leukaemias.

4. Prezygotic cancers and leukaemias are biased in favour of primitive cell types and may have a familial incidence. Post-zygotic cancers and leukaemias are biased in favour of mature cell types and have no familial incidence.

5. Individuals who develop prezygotic leukaemias have no normal leucocytes and therefore have an exceptionally low resistance to infections. The pedigrees of index cases have not been fully elucidated because the equivalent disease in relatives may take several forms—for example, leucopenia, anaemia, low resistance to infections, and leukaemia.

6. In childhood the maximum incidence of prezygotic leukaemias is earlier than the maximum incidence of prenatal leukaemias.

7. The recent increase in childhood leukaemias is a consequence of the falling death-rate for pneumonia and related diseases, and is due to prezygotic leukaemias.

* The numbering of references in this excerpt has been changed from the original in order to agree with the numeration of references in the present volume.

The concept of cancer being a process of two or more stages is of course not new (*vide* 1, 2, 3), and induction and promotion have been invoked in experimental studies (85). For instance, coal tar derivatives painted on the skin are reckoned to induce malignant change which does not manifest itself for some long time after; but the cancer can be promoted to appear much earlier by an application of croton oil, which itself is no inducing agent.

On this working hypothesis the very much commoner variety of childhood leukemia is in no wise attributable to diagnostic radiography of the mother during pregnancy, and the inducing agent, physical, chemical or spontaneous, is unknown. Only in the second variety, where death before the age of 5 years is unusual, is radiation of the unborn fetus or the recently born infant specifically incriminated.

Even this association is not generally accepted. The survey of Stewart and her group was retrospective, a large number of established cases of leukemia and other malignancies of childhood being taken and followed backward. This process needs a selected population for comparison as control. The selection of these control populations inevitably involves some arbitrary decisions which may bias the comparison. Moreover, the method involves memory of the subjects interviewed, and individuals are notoriously fallible at remembering. Other surveys of this retrospective type have been made in the U.S.A., notably by Ford *et al.* (86) whose findings were substantially in accord with Stewart's. In smaller series the association was not significantly different from that of chance (87, 88). The alternative survey to the retrospective is the prospective, such as that carried out by Court Brown, Doll, and Bradford Hill (89), where no association was detected. The *British Medical Journal*, reviewing in a leading article at the time, summed up:

Whatever may be the correct explanation of observations accepted as facts, there are other observations which still require validation. From the practical aspect the most important was that of Alice Stewart and her colleagues [82*]. From a retrospective statistical survey of cases of

---

* The numbering of references in this excerpt has been changed from the original in order to agree with the numeration of references in the present volume.

malignancy in childhood, they derived an association of malignancy with X-irradiation during foetal life, suggesting that such irradiated children had twice the normal chance of dying from malignancy before the age of 10. In the opening pages of the *Journal* this week Dr. W. M. Court Brown, Dr. R. Doll, and Professor A. Bradford Hill [89] review what confirmation or lack of it there has been from other surveys and give their own statistics to date of a prospective survey of children who had been exposed while still *in utero* to X-rays applied for diagnostic purposes. There were 9 deaths from leukaemia before the age of 14 instead of the expected 10.5 from the group of 40,000-odd children in the survey. Mr. T. L. T. Lewis [90] also reports the results of an investigation into this problem . . . obtaining a negative result from an analysis of records from Queen Charlotte's Hospital, London.

These figures illustrate the difficulty of this type of statistical investigation. The death-rates from leukaemia even in a period of 10 years or so are small, so that differences between the control and investigated groups must in absolute numbers be small, and significance rests on the relativity. Retrospective surveys are suspect because they depend on past history, and human memory is fallible. Prospective surveys may suffer from the failure to identify some real consequences of the act investigated; but in general more confidence is engendered by the prospective survey.

In the present context the reader will not find scientific disproof of either hypothesis. It is possible here only to attempt a judicious opinion. The results of Court Brown and his colleagues suggest that, if leukaemia is induced in children by diagnostic irradiation as practised in the respective hospitals at the relevant time, it was too infrequent to be detectable by an investigation of manageable size. From the much larger numbers of cases of malignancy in childhood which Stewart and her colleagues were able to select, we must conclude that, if diagnostic irradiation had the carcinogenic effect their statistics indicated, the capacity of X-rays for the production of leukaemia was 10 times or more greater in the foetus than at any other age.*

What the clinician needs to know is: Will the use of diagnostic X-rays on the abdomen of the pregnant women or the withholding of them lead to the greater human suffering? There seems to have been no published appreciation of this problem. The Committee on Radiological Hazards to Patients [91] has evaluated the situation for mass miniature radiog-

---

* Brian MacMahon of Harvard (personal communication) has now completed a larger prospective survey involving 700,000 children to estimate that cancer mortality of the X-rayed is 1.4 times that of the non-X-rayed. This value would be within the error of both the prospective survey of Court Brown *et al.* and the retrospective survey of Stewart *et al.*

raphy and concluded that the benefits of early identification of curable
pulmonary disease far outweigh the disadvantages of the calculated
numbers of cases of induced leukaemia. The answer for obstetric radiology
rests on the provision of quantitative data by the obstetrician of how
much the recent reduction in maternal and foetal morbidity and mortality
has been attributable to the information derived from X-rays. Against
this can be set the possible numbers of malformations and neoplasms
induced by the radiation. On radiobiological grounds it seems likely that
the hazard is preponderantly from radiation given to the embryo in the
first trimester. There are thus sound reasons for advising delay of diagnostic irradiation when possible.

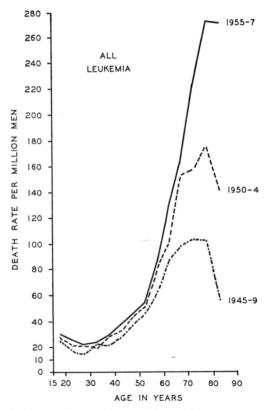

FIG. 23.—Mortality from all forms of leukemia among men at different
ages (from 15 years upward) in England and Wales in 1945–49, 1950–54,
and 1955–57. (From W. M. Court Brown and R. Doll, in *Brit. Med. J.*,
1 [1959]: 1063, Fig. 1.)

Adults.—The recorded death rates during various periods in Britain are given for adults as well as children in Table 1, provided by Court Brown and Doll (92). They had also reviewed the subject of adult leukemia in 1959 (93), and from this paper Figures 23–26 are taken. These figures give the death rates for 3 recent periods

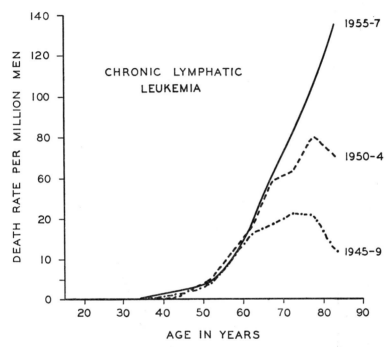

FIG. 24.—Estimated mortality from chronic lymphatic leukemia among men at different ages (from 15 years upward) in England and Wales in 1945–49, 1950–54, and 1955–57. (From W. M. Court Brown and R. Doll, in *Brit. Med. J.*, 1 [1959]: 1063, Fig. 2.)

versus age according to the particular types of leukemia—all types, chronic lymphatic, chronic myeloid, and acute leukemia. The rise in all cases between the first and latest period is patent. However, the opinion is expressed that the rises noted in the elderly are mainly an expression of improvements in diagnosis and certification, for the same phenomenon is seen for cancer of the lung and gastric ulcer while there is a large decrease in deaths certified as

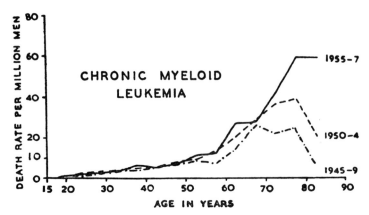

FIG. 25.—Estimated mortality from chronic myeloid leukemia among men at different ages (from 15 years upward) in England and Wales in 1945–49, 1950–54, and 1955–57. (From W. M. Court Brown and R. Doll, in *Brit. Med. J.*, 1 [1959]: 1063, Fig. 3.)

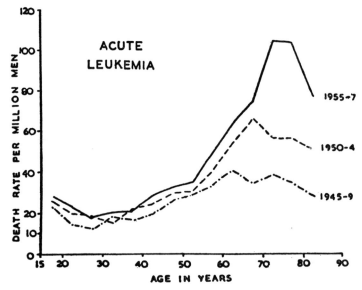

FIG. 26.—Estimated mortality from acute leukemia among men at different ages (from 15 years upward) in England and Wales in 1945–49, 1950–54, and 1955–57. (From W. M. Court Brown and R. Doll, in *Brit. Med. J.*, 1 [1959]: 1063, Fig. 4.)

due to senility. If the over 65's are excluded for this reason, the only real increase appears to be in the death rate from acute leukemia affecting men and women equally.

The question arises, "Is this increase in acute leukemia of adults due in any way to ionizing radiation, or is it due to the introduction of one or more other leukemogenic agents in our environment?" The answer cannot be given categorically at the present time. What we can say is that we know far more about radiation as a leukemogenic agent than about the others, but this should not lead us into the trap into which the uncritical fall of attributing all leukemia to radiation—natural or man made.

There can be little doubt that the pattern of mortality is altering with time. There can similarly be no doubt that the patterns of life and environment are also altering. It is logical, though not necessarily true, to relate the former to the latter of these phenomena; but it is not even logical to consider the increasing uses of radiation as the only environmental change of potential leukemogenic importance. The incidence of cancer of the lung has increased concomitantly with that of leukemia, but radiation is not invoked as a cause for that. Instead carcinogens in cigarette smoke are blamed with some justification from statistics. Cigarette smoking is also blamed as a part cause for the rise in reported coronary thrombosis. I have no doubt a case could be made for smoking as a causative factor in leukemia, particularly if Alice Stewart is right that many of the childhood leukemias can be traced to prezygotic influences.

Now is not the time in which to dilate on all the other alterations in environment of the present century which could directly or indirectly affect the present patterns of mortality. We may merely note that correlations of a qualitative nature exist. The task of today is to make measurements for quantitative assessments. As far as radiation is concerned, a start has been made. Over the last few years national figures are emerging for population radiation doses received from medical procedures—diagnosis and therapy. In the United Kingdom the Adrian Committee (94) has recently reported that "the total annual genetic dose from all medical radiology in 1957 has been calculated to be 19.3 mr per person."

This is a valuable figure to have available, but let it be noted that the genetically effective dose is much easier to derive than the leukemogenically effective dose, for the germ cells are concentrated in a small circumscribed volume of the individual. The hemopoietic cells are widely distributed, so that for any radiological exposure many will be in the radiation field but most will not be. We do not yet know how to allow for this factor.

In other fields, too, measurements are being made. For example, atmospheric pollution is known to affect morbidity and mortality, including that from some cancers. Given reasonably reliable statistics of environmental factors, the next generation should be able to relate them to vital statistics with more confidence than ours.

HUMAN LEUKEMIA AND RADIATION

It is appropriate at this stage to review this subject—briefly, because it has been done many times recently. The National Academy of Sciences (95) in the U.S.A., the Medical Research Council (25) in Britain, and the United Nations Scientific Committee on the Effects of Atomic Radiation (21) have all said their say and so have a number of individuals (96, 97, 98).

1. *Radiologists.* It has been noted earlier that in the U.S.A. fairly definitely and in the U.K. only doubtfully, because of the smaller numbers available for analysis, there has been a recorded incidence of leukemia higher than in comparable populations. However the doses of radiation to which the radiologists of that generation were exposed is not known with any certainty and can only be guessed. Now that occupationally received doses are being recorded more or less faithfully, it should be possible to reassess this hazard sometime in the future.

The distribution of radiation dose in radiologists must have been non-uniform but for practical purposes can be taken as to the whole body.

2. *Atomic bomb survivors.* Within a few years of the explosion of the atomic bombs over Hiroshima and Nagasaki, an increased mortality from leukemia was suspected. Reliable figures of this mortality are now available (99, 100). In Hiroshima the incidence

of leukemia per year in survivors of the explosion is rather small in absolute numbers (Fig. 27). There appeared to be a maximum in 1952 with a subsequent decline, but the latest data do not give grounds for postulating any simple relationship. In relative numbers the incidence of leukemia per million per year is high for

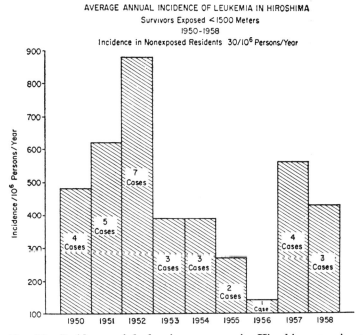

FIG. 27.—Incidence of leukemia per year in Hiroshima survivors. (From R. Heyssel and A. B. Brill, in *Radioactivity in Man*, ed. G. R. Meneely [Springfield, Ill., 1961], Fig. 1. Courtesy of Charles C Thomas, Publisher.)

those who were exposed near to the hypocenter, and there is a linear decline of this incidence with increasing distance from the hypocenter (Fig. 28). The exact doses of radiation received by individuals is a matter for much calculation and recalculation. Both neutrons and γ-rays were involved, and there is internal evidence from the data that shielding must have been quite important but obviously difficult to calculate. One can only say that there

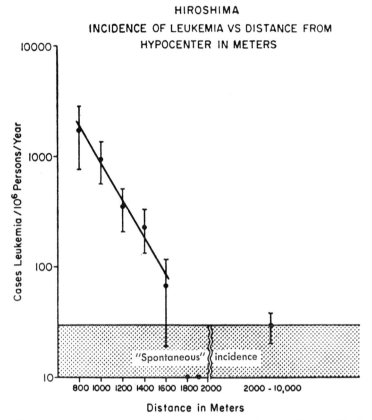

FIG. 28.—Distance from the hypocenter related to incidence of leukemia—Hiroshima. (From R. Heyssel and A. B. Brill, in *Radioactivity in Man*, ed. G. R. Meneely [Springfield, Ill., 1961], Fig. 2. Courtesy of Charles C Thomas, Publisher.)

must have been a rough correlation of radiation dose with distance from the hypocenter.

Again, the distribution of radiation dose in the individuals exposed will have been non-uniform, but the whole body must have been irradiated.

3. *Patients with ankylosing spondylitis.* The first report of the Medical Research Council (101) on the *Hazards to Man of Nuclear and Allied Radiations* reported a study of the delayed effects of

radiotherapy of such patients. This has been elaborated by Court Brown and Doll (102). The records of 13,000 patients were scrutinized and some 30 or more cases of leukemia identified. Since the radiation was given as X-ray therapy, the doses given and their distribution are known with some precision. However, as the whole body was not irradiated but only the parts affected by disease, a considerable volume it is true, there are difficulties in deciding what dose to use as the yardstick—the integral dose to the whole body or the maximum or mean dose in spinal bone marrow. When the last was used, there was a linear relation between this dose and the subsequent incidence of leukemia.

Wise (103) has reviewed the detail of this series to conclude that "the probability of onset (i.e. leukemia) is found to increase suddenly to a maximum in the fourth year after the inducing radiation. . . . The analysis in general confirms that leukemia can be caused by X-rays but throws doubt on the assumed linear-dose response relationships, which depend upon assuming a uniform distribution of latent periods."

Faber (104) in Denmark has also made very extensive study not only of radiotherapy but of diagnostic X-ray exposure and the relation to leukemia.

4. *Patients (children) with thymic enlargement.* These subjects have also been mentioned in passing. Hemplemann (97), who has played an active part in this research, has summarized the evidence in an excellent general review, "Epidemological Studies of Leukemia in Persons Exposed to Ionizing Radiation." The incidence of leukemia and other cancers were increased in certain treated groups reported from Rochester. Contrariwise, from other centers, while no increase of leukemia has been reported, an increase in carcinoma of thyroid was evident. Further studies according to Hemplemann are required to elucidate the importance or otherwise of so-called thymic enlargement on the one hand and of radiation factors, like size of field irradiated, on the other hand, since these varied between the centers reporting.

In series such as these, the doses received by individuals are well documented since this is therapy. However "in the nine cases observed in children treated for thymic enlargement, there was no obvious correlation between dose and incidence." Since the radiation given is to a local area only, the same problems arise as in the patients with ankylosing spondylitis; what is the true yardstick?

Another and earlier review which has been more than usually read and quoted is that by E. B. Lewis (96), a geneticist of great renown, "Leukemia and Ionizing Radiation." As a geneticist he naturally brought something of a new look to this problem, accenting as might be expected the quantitative aspects that could be derived by considering leukemia as a manifestation of somatic mutation. Then, by examination of the data on series of human subjects where induction of leukemia by radiation is generally accepted, he calculated in each case the probability of inducing leukemia per individual per rad per year. The following table is abridged from Lewis:

TABLE 2

Source	Region Irradiated	"Best Estimate of Probability"
Atom bomb survivors............	Whole body	2×10^{-6}
Ankylosing spondylitis patients....	Spine	1×10^{-6}
Thymic enlargement patients.....	Chest	1×10^{-6}
Radiologists...................	Partial to whole body	2×10^{-6}

The relatively small scatter of "best estimates" is remarkable considering the variety of the groups. The atom bomb survivors had 1 exposure to mixed neutron and γ-radiations: the ankylosing spondylitis patients had multiple exposures to X-ray therapy to spine and other joints for the relief of pain and immobility; the thymic enlargement patients were children given 1 or more therapeutic exposures to reduce the size of an allegedly enlarged thymus gland; and the radiologists received variable exposures over the course of a working lifetime. On the other hand all the data are derived from subjects who received their irradiation, single or multiple, usually the latter, at a high dose-rate. What Lewis did, and which I have not copied, was to include in his table another group—spontaneous incidence of leukemia (Brooklyn, N.Y.)—who are taken to have received only natural background radiation throughout life at the very low dose-rate of 0.1–0.2 rad per year: the best estimate is listed as 2×10^{-6} like the others in the table. But the value of 2×10^{-6} was not calculated from the data as for the other groups; it was merely adopted. By its adoption and multiplication with the average age in years of Brooklyners—33.7 years and radiation dose per year of 0.1–0.2 rad—a mortality rate of 7 to 13 cases per million per year due to background radiation was deduced, or some 10–20 per cent of the observed rate of 65 cases per million per year.

The very great merit of Lewis' work is not the derivation of numbers, no matter how convincing they may look, but in its challenge to others to test his hypothesis. Since its publication, evidence has now accrued that among spondylitics the age of the irradiated subject is a factor for the reckoning—the older the subject the greater probability of leukemia supervening; that in the spondylitics and perhaps atom bomb survivors the probability of leukemia reaches a maximum after some 5 years and then declines; that in experimentally induced leukemias of the mouse dose-rate is a most important factor. All these points are very much against the basic hypothesis of Lewis of a linear relation of dose to leukemic effect irrespective of time. Unhappily it is not possible to claim for Lewis's work as others have done, "It is now possible to calculate —within narrow limits—how many deaths from leukemia will result in any population from any increase in fall-out or other source of radiation" (105). This is just wishful journalese.

The burning questions to me are not what are the numbers of leukemia to be expected from atom bombs or radiotherapy, but what is to be expected from natural background (and any man-made addition to it) and from medical diagnostic radiology. Furthermore, to obtain estimates of these, I believe it is wrong to go to atom bombs, where the radiations are qualitatively different and, more important, the dose-rate outstandingly different.

Pursuing much the same line of thought, Court Brown *et al.* (106) made a survey of leukemia in Scotland, since parts of Scotland, notably Aberdeenshire and the City of Aberdeen, are rich in granite, which gives a rather higher natural background of radiation than sedimentary rocks. Spiers made the detailed measurements of radiation doses, which indicated that average doses in bone marrow should be 80, 86, and 101 *mrad*. per year in Edinburgh, Dundee, and Aberdeen respectively. Thus, while the background radiation out of doors in Aberdeen is twice that of Edinburgh, the difference is much less when all the relevant factors are taken into account. If according to Lewis' speculations natural background radiation were to be responsible for some 10–20 per cent of natural leukemia, one would not expect a 20 per cent difference in background to show an effect in a city of less than 200,000 people like Aberdeen. Nevertheless, the observed results were very revealing. Over an 18-year period the death rate from leukemia was nearly half as much again as the national average for Scotland. Thus either Lewis underestimated the effect of background by a hundredfold or more, or background radiation is apparently 100 or more times less important than other factors. The authors incline to the latter view stressing that real, as distinct from apparent, incidence is very hard to determine because of variability in "case-finding."

Thus the problems in real life are much the same as the difficulties discussed earlier for laboratory experiments. The wider the net is cast, the more variables and imponderables enter into the final analysis. Many have hoped that somewhere in the world one would find populations larger than that of Aberdeen living in areas of higher natural background, so that the influence of background on leukemia and similar conditions could be measured. In fact such conditions have been identified in Kerala in India. Unhappily no vital statistics are available for this region, and only recently have good physical measurements been begun. Now, one wonders, even if facilities can be provided for the collection of the medical statistics, will the material be sufficiently homogeneous to provide a reliable answer?

For the present, all that I would be prepared to say about the effects of natural background on the incidence of leukemia would be that the subject is *sub judice*. The human observations, as far as they go, suggest that other factors are much more important. The experiments on mice indicate that, to get readily measurable increases in the incidence of murine leukemia, the additions to background have to be more than one thousand times the background, but these figures are not to be translated directly to man.

Medical diagnostic radiology is also a subject meet for consideration. Faber's (104) inquiries in Denmark lead us to the conclusion that it cannot be neglected as a cause of leukemia: by the same token we can say that any effect it has had in the past must be marginal only. We are thus left with a value judgment. Has diagnostic radiology provided more benefits than distress—and the balanced opinion has so far always been yes, though it is often difficult to express this as numbers in the style of a profit-and-loss account. It is not likely to become easier as far as the loss side is concerned.

What we can say is that the hazard has been identified, so that an increasing effort is being made at all levels—by manufacturers of equipment, by physicians and radiologists—to reduce the dose delivered per necessary exposure. Although many more radiological exposures are made today than, say, a generation ago, measured by the gross sale of film, nevertheless the total dose delivered today may well be less, due to improvements already made. Now there are means whereby the doses delivered can be measured and a running check kept on this factor rather than on film used. However, we have already indicated that we still require to develop appropriate weighting factors for exposures affecting different organs and parts of the body.

Certainly our present concern, probably rightly, is mostly with radiography of the pregnant woman, for then two individuals are being exposed at the same time, the fetus probably totally if the mother's abdomen and pelvis are the subject for examination. It is a general radiobiological axiom that dividing tissues are particularly radiosensitive, and there is good evidence of the radiosensitivity of the mammalian fetus, particularly in the early stages when tissues are differentiating. The work of Stewart suggests that, particularly at this stage and even later in fetal development up till birth, irradiation may be a factor in inducing leukemia subsequently in childhood; but the uncertainties due to the variable results of different groups have been noted. According to Stewart (*vide supra*) (82) children having been irradiated as fetuses *in utero* have twice the chance of dying of malignant disease before the age of 10. The X-ray doses given to the subjects of this survey are not of course known. At the present time the average dose might be about 1 rad; at that time it may well have been up to some 5 times greater. If 5 rads doubled the natural death rate from malignancy in children up to the age of 10 (1:1200 according to Stewart), this is equivalent to an average induction rate per rad of 16×10^{-6} per year. About half of the childhood malignancies are leukemias, so on this reckoning the *minimum* value for induction of leukemia would be 8×10^{-6} per rad per year.

For one who has no vested interest for or against radiation, the matter can be expressed in this way. Of the children dying of leukemia and other malignant diseases before the age of 10, 87 per cent were not irradiated as fetuses *in utero*, so that for the vast majority this hazard is an irrelevancy. This receives confirmation from Stewart (83) who believes that most leukemias in children (and I infer that this means more than 3 out of 4) are determined before conception. So in the remaining 13 per cent who were irradiated as fetuses, the irradiation was also an irrelevancy in about 9, leaving about 4 per cent in whom the irradiation might have played a part. While not losing sight of this possible 4 per cent, we should concentrate our effort on trying to understand the 96 per cent—which may be 100 per cent.

References

1. Armitage, P., and Doll, R. Brit. J. Cancer, **8:** 1. 1954.
2. ———, and ———. Brit. J. Cancer, **11:** 161. 1957.
3. Sacher, G. *In:* The Delayed Effects of Whole Body Radiation, ed. B. B. Watson, p. 3. Johns Hopkins Press, Baltimore, Md. 1960.

4. NEARY, G. J. Nature (Lond.), **187**: 10. 1960.
5. MEDAWAR, P. B. An Unsolved Problem of Biology. H. K. Lewis, London. 1952.
6. GOMPERTZ, B. Phil. Trans., **115**: 513. 1825.
7. STREHLER, B. L. Quart. Rev. Biol., **34**: 117, 1959.
8. SACHER, G. Radiology, **67**: 250. 1956.
9. MULLER, H. J. J. Cell. Comp. Physiol., **35** (Supp. 1): 9. 1950.
10. HENSHAW, P. S. Radiology, **69**: 30. 1957.
11. FAILLA, G. Radiology, **69**: 23. 1957.
12. YOCKEY, H. P. *In:* Symposium on Information Theory in Biology, ed. H. P. YOCKEY, R. L. PLATZMAN, and H. QUASTLER, p. 297. Pergamon Press, London. 1958.
13. SZILARD, L. Proc. Nat. Acad. Sci., **45**: 30. 1959.
14. SPEAR, F. G. *In:* Radiations and Living Cells, p. 2. Chapman & Hall, London. 1953.
15. MARCH, H. C. Radiology, **43**: 275. 1944. Amer. J. Med. Sci., **220**: 282. 1950.
16. HENSHAW, P. S., and HAWKINS, J. W. J. Nat. Cancer Inst., **4**: 339. 1944.
17. DUBLIN, L. I., and SPIEGELMAN, M. J. Amer. Med. Assn., **134**: 1211. 1947.
18. WARREN, S. J. Amer. Med. Assn., **162**: 464. 1956.
19. SELTSER, R., and SARTWELL, P. E. J. Amer. Med. Assn., **166**: 585. 1958.
20. COURT BROWN, W. M., and DOLL, R. *In:* Progress in Nuclear Energy VII Medical Sciences 2, ed. J. BUGHER, J. COURSAGET, and J. F. LOUTIT, p. 21. Pergamon Press, London. 1959.
21. UNITED NATIONS SCIENTIFIC COMMITTEE. The Effects of Atomic Radiation. New York. 1958.
22. LINDOP, P. and ROTBLAT, J. Nature (Lond.), **189**: 645, 1961.
23. ———, Proc. Roy. Soc. Ser. B., **154**: 332, 350. 1961.
24. MOLE, R. H. Nature (Lond.), **180**: 456, 1957.
25. MEDICAL RESEARCH COUNCIL. Hazards to Man of Nuclear and Allied Radiations. Cmnd. 1225. H.M.S.O., London. 1960.
26. INTERNATIONAL COMMISSION ON RADIOLOGICAL PROTECTION. Recommendations. Pergamon Press, London. 1959.
27. NEARY, G. J.; MUNSON, R. J.; and MOLE, R. H. Chronic Radiation Hazards: An experimental study with fast neutrons. Pergamon Press, London. 1957.
28. LORENZ, E.; JACOBSON, L. O.; HESTON, W. E.; SHIMKIN, M.; ESCHENBRENNER, A. B.; DERINGER, M. K.; DONIGER, J.; and SCHWEISTHAL, R. *In:* Biological Effects of External X and Gam-

ma Radiation, ed. R. E. ZIRKLE, NNES IV–22B, p. 24. McGraw-Hill, New York. 1954.

29. JONES, H. B. *In:* Advances in Biological and Medical Physics, ed. C. A. TOBIAS and J. H. LAWRENCE, p. 281. Academic Press, New York. 1956.
30. MOLE, R. H. J. Nat. Cancer Inst., 15: 907. 1955.
31. RUSSELL, W. L., and RUSSELL, L. B. *In:* Progress in Nuclear Energy VI Biological Sciences 2, ed. J. C. BUGHER, J. COURT SAGET, and J. F. LOUTIT, p. 179. Pergamon Press, London. 1959.
32. UPTON, A. C.; KIMBALL, A. W.; FURTH, J.; CHRISTENBERRY, K. W.; and BENEDICT, W. H. Cancer Res., 20 (No. 8, Part 2): 110. 1960.
33. KAPLAN, H. S., and BROWN, M. B. J. Nat. Cancer Inst., 13: 185. 1952.
34. MOLE, R. H. *In:* Progress in Radiobiology, ed. J. S. MITCHELL, B. E. HOLMES, and C. L. SMITH, p. 468. Oliver and Boyd, Edinburgh. 1956.
35. KAPLAN, H. S. J. Nat. Cancer Inst., 11: 83. 1950.
36. MOLE, R. H. In press.
37. HENRY, H. F. Report K1470 Union Carbide Nuclear Co. Off. Tech. Serv. U.S. Dept. Commerce., Washington, D.C. 1961.
38. CARLSON, L. D., and JACKSON, B. Radiat. Res., 11: 509. 1959.
39. ELLERMAN, V., and BANG, O. Zentralbl. Bact. I. Orig., 46: 595. 1908.
40. ROUS, P. J. Exp. Med., 12: 696. 1910.
41. BITTNER, J. J. Science, 84: 162. 1936.
42. GROSS, L. Proc. Soc. Exp. Biol. (N.Y.), 76: 27. 1951.
43. STEWART, S. E.; EDDY, B. E.; and STANTON, M. F. *In:* Canadian Cancer Conference 3, ed. R. W. BEGG, p. 287. Academic Press, New York. 1958.
44. FORD, C. E.; JACOBS, P. A.; and LAJTHA, L. G. Nature (Lond.), 181: 1565. 1958.
45. FORD, C. E.; HAMERTON, J. L.; and MOLE, R. H. J. Cell. Comp. Physiol., 52 (Supp. 1): 235. 1958.
46. BAIKIE, A. G.; JACOBS, P. A.; McBRIDE, J. A.; and TOUGH, I. M. Brit. Med. J., 1: 1564. 1961.
47. NOWELL, P. C., and HUNGERFORD, D. A. J. Nat. Cancer Inst., 25: 85. 1960.
48. BOND, V. P.; CRONKITE, E. P.; FLIEDNER, T. N.; and SCHORK, P. Science, 128: 202. 1958.
49. LOUTIT, J. F. Ann. N.Y. Acad. Sci., 88: 122. 1960.
50. POPP, R. A. Proc. Soc. Exp. Biol. (N.Y.), 104: 722. 1960.
51. LAJTHA, L. G., and OLIVER, R. Haemopoiesis, CIBA Foundation Symposium, p. 289. London. 1960.

52. BARNES, D. W. H.; FORD, C. E.; and LOUTIT, J. F. Sang, 30: 762. 1959.

53. TOUGH, I. M.; COURT BROWN, W. M.; BAIKIE, A. G.; BUCKTON, K. E.; HARNDEN, D. G.; JACOBS, P.; KING, M.; and McBRIDE, J. A. Lancet, 1: 411. 1961.

54. CARTER, T. C.; LYON, M. F.; and PHILLIPS, R. J. S. J. Genet., 53: 154. 1955.

55. FORD, C. E.; HAMERTON, J. L.; BARNES, D. W. H.; and LOUTIT, J. F. Nature (Lond.), 177: 452. 1956.

56. TJIO, J. H., and LEVAN, A. Hereditas, 42: 1. 1956.

57. FORD, C. E., and HAMERTON, J. L. Nature (Lond.), 178: 1020. 1956.

58. DENVER CLASSIFICATION. Supp. Cerebral Palsy Bull. 2, No. 3. 1960.

59. JACOBS, P. A.; COURT BROWN, W. M., and DOLL, R. *Nature* (Lond.), 191: 1178. 1961.

60. NOWELL, P. C., and HUNGERFORD, D. A. Lancet, 1: 113. 1960.

61. FLOREY, H. W. *In:* General Pathology, 2d ed., p. 118. Lloyd Luke, London. 1958.

62. METCALF, D. *In:* Canadian Cancer Conference 3, ed. R. W. BEGG, p. 351. Academic Press, New York. 1959.

63. KAPLAN, H. S.; HIRSCH, B. B.; and BROWN, M. B. Cancer Res., 16: 434. 1956.

64. LAW, L. W., and POTTER, M. Proc. Nat. Acad. Sci., 42: 160. 1956.

65. BARNES, D. W. H.; FORD, C. E.; ILBERY, P. L. T.; JONES, K. W.; and LOUTIT, J. F. Acta Un. Internat. Contre Cancer, 15 (Nos. 3–4) · 544 1959.

66. GROSS, L. Proc. Soc. Exp. Biol. (N.Y.), 100: 102. 1959.

67. KAPLAN, H. S. *In:* Phenomena of Tumor Viruses. National Cancer Institute Monograph No. 4, p. 141. 1960.

68. GROSS, L. Acta haematol., 23: 259, 1960.

69. BURNET, F. M., and FENNER, F. The Production of Antibodies, 2d ed. Macmillan, Melbourne. 1949.

70. GROSS, L. Acta haematol., 13: 13. 1955.

71. SHAPIRO, F.; MARTINEZ, C.; SMITH, J. M.; and GOOD, R. A. Proc. Soc. Exp. Biol. (N.Y.), 106: 472. 1961.

72. KAPLAN, H. S. Cancer Res., 14: 535 1954.

73. LOUTIT, J. F. *In:* Advances in Radiobiology, ed. G. C. DE HEVESY, A. G. FORSSBERG, and J. D. ABBATT, p. 388. Oliver and Boyd, Edinburgh. 1957.

74. MICKLEM, H. S., and FORD, C. E. Transplant. Bull., 26: 436. 1960.

75. ———. Personal communication.

76. FICHTELIUS, K. E. *In:* Haemopoiesis, CIBA Foundation Symposium, p. 204. J. & A. Churchill, London. 1960.

77. MOLE, R. II. Brit. Med. Bull., 14: 174. 1958.
78. MOLE, R. H. Brit. J. Radiol., 32: 497. 1959.
79. UPTON, A. C.; WOLFF, F. F.; FURTH, J.; and KIMBALL, A. W. Cancer Res., 18: 842. 1958.
80. GRAFFI, A. Ann. N.Y. Acad. Sci., 68: 540. 1957.
81. WOOD, E. E. Brit. Med. J., 1: 1760, 1960.
82. STEWART, ALICE; WEBB. J.; and HEWITT, D. Brit. Med. J., 1: 1495. 1958.
83. STEWART, ALICE. Brit. Med. J., 1: 452. 1961.
84. LEJEUNE, J.; GAUTHER, M.; and TURPIN, R. C. R. Acad. Sci., 248: 602. 1959.
85. BERENBLUM, I., *In:* General Pathology, 2d ed., ed. H. W. FLOREY, p. 513. Lloyd Luke, London. 1958.
86. FORD, D. D.; PATERSON, J. C. S.; and TREUTING, W. L. J. Nat. Cancer Inst., 22: 1093. 1959.
87. KAPLAN, H. S. Amer. J. Roentgenol., 80: 696. 1958.
88. POLHEMUS, D. W., and KOCH, R. Pediatrics, 23: 453. 1959.
89. COURT BROWN, W. M.; DOLL, R.; and BRADFORD HILL, A. Brit. Med. J., 2: 1539. 1960.
90. LEWIS, T. L. T. Brit. Med. J., 2: 1551. 1960.
91. MINISTRY OF HEALTH. Radiological Hazards to Patients. Interim Report. H.M.S.O., London. 1959.
92. COURT BROWN, W. M., and DOLL, R. Appendix. *In:* Medical Research Council Hazards to Man of Nuclear and Allied Radiations. Cmnd. 1225. H.M.S.O., London. 1960.
93. COURT BROWN, W. M., and DOLL, R. Brit. Med. J., 1: 1063, 1959.
94. MINISTRY OF HEALTH. Radiological Hazards to Patients. 2d Report. H.M.S.O., London. 1960.
95. NATIONAL ACADEMY OF SCIENCES—NATIONAL RESEARCH COUNCIL. Publication 875. Effects of Ionizing Radiation on the Human Hemopoietic System. Washington, D.C. 1961.
96. LEWIS, E. B. Science, 125: 965, 1957.
97. HEMPELMANN, L. H. Cancer Res., 20: 18, 1960.
98. HEYSSEL, R. M., and BRILL, A. B. *In:* Radioactivity in Man, ed. G. R. MENEELY, p. 266. C C Thomas, Springfield, Ill. 1961.
99. LANGE, R. D.; MALONEY, W. C.; and YAMAWAKI, T. Blood, 9: 574, 1954.
100. HEYSSEL, R. M.; BRILL, A. B.; WOODBURY, L. A.; NISHIMURA, E. T.; GHOSE, T.; HOSHINO, T.; and YAMASAKI, M. Blood, 15: 313. 1960.
101. MEDICAL RESEARCH COUNCIL. The Hazards to Man of Nuclear and Allied Radiations. Cmd. 9780. H.M.S.O., London. 1956.

102. COURT BROWN, W. M., and DOLL, R. Spec. Rep. Series Medical Research Council, No. 295. H.M.S.O., London. 1957.
103. WISE, M. E. Health Physics, 4: 250. 1961.
104. FABER, M. Nord. Med., 59: 839. 1958.
105. SCIENCE, 125: 963. 1957. Leading article.
106. COURT BROWN, W. M.; DOLL, R.; SPIERS, F. W.; DUFFY, B. J.; and McHUGH, M. J. Brit. Med. J., 1: 1753. 1960.

CHAPTER THREE

STRONTIUM 90

Radioactive Strontium Isotopes

In the fission of uranium 235 or plutonium 239 several isotopes of strontium are formed as fission products. Two of them, strontium 89 and strontium 90, particularly the latter, deserve special consideration because of their long radioactive half-lifes—50 days and 30 years respectively. The other fission-product strontium isotopes have quite short half-lifes and thus are relatively of little consequence as biological hazards. Yet another radioactive isotope, strontium 85, is not a fission product (in practice it is produced by special techniques in cyclotrons) but like strontium 89 is a medium-lived radionucleide with a half-time of 65 days. It is preferred to strontium 89 for experimental studies since, being a pure γ-ray emitter, it leads to a less concentrated radiation dose in bone than the β-particle emitter strontium 89; and, since a large fraction of its γ-rays pass through the tissues overlying the skeleton, its activity can be measured by placing the experimental animal or man in a "whole-body counter." Its retention in the body can thus be measured directly and speedily, whereas retention of the β-emitting strontium 89 or strontium 90 can usually be measured only by the indirect means of subtracting what has been excreted up to any particular time from what had been administered; this is a time-consuming job and subject to considerable experimental error.

THE HAZARDS FROM FISSION-PRODUCT STRONTIUM

From the earliest times after the discovery of nuclear fission, the hazard arising from the long-lived fission products was appreciated. The reason is obvious. The element strontium is a chemical analogue of calcium, as also are barium and radium. All these elements would be expected to behave, if they gained entry into the body, in much the same way as calcium. Indeed the dangers of ingesting radium, as an occupational hazard in the luminizing industry, were well known. In the previous two decades a substantial number of deaths and diseases had been recorded in luminizers from retention of radium in their bones. This led to severe anemia in the most acute cases, due to the effect on the blood-forming tissue in the bone marrow, destruction of bone (necrosis) with spontaneous fracture in less acute cases, and not infrequently malignant bone tumor (osteosarcoma) with retained amounts of a few micrograms of radium.

To estimate the hazard from the radioactive fission products strontium 89 and strontium 90, one requires to know first the metabolic behavior of strontium—its distribution and turnover—compared with radium and of both compared with calcium, and second the comparative radiotoxicity of β-particle-emitting radioactive strontium fission products and the α-particle-emitting radium and its complicated system of radioactive decay products.

The metabolic behavior of radioactive strontium (Sr^{85} and Sr^{89}) was extensively investigated in experimental animals in the University of California at Berkeley by Pecher (1) and then Hamilton (2). Complementary work was carried out in Chicago. The most notable contribution of the workers of Chicago, both in the early days of nuclear energy and now, however, has been in the field of radiotoxicology. Our current estimates of hazard are based almost completely on the work of Austin Brues, Miriam Finkel, and their associates, working with experimental animals given strontium 89 or strontium 90 (3, 4), and the toxicological studies in man, contaminated with radium, of Marinelli, Hasterlik, and their groups (5, 6). This latter work has extended and refined the earlier surveys of Martland (7) and Evans (8).

Recent Research Programs in
Strontium Metabolism

The laboratory which I have the honor to direct has placed its effort into the study of the metabolic behavior of strontium in man. Work on experimental animals is invaluable as a first approach, and, if all species investigated gave identical results, these could be translated to the assessment of the human hazard with considerable confidence. Not unnaturally, however, different species of animal show different patterns of behavior. The small rodents, mice and rats, the most convenient animals to use in the laboratory for many purposes, in fact have a rather different bone structure. They also have a very much intensified general metabolism and heat output per unit mass because of their large surface/mass ratio. Some of the larger animals which have been investigated, cows, goats, and sheep, being ruminants and vegetarians, have quite a different digestive apparatus from our own. Ultimately, therefore, one requires specific information on man over and above the basic data that one can acquire from other mammals.

The first exercise of my colleague, Harrison (9), was to see what could be learned from the administration to normal human subjects of stable strontium either by mouth or intravenously. This stable strontium is present in all mineral sources of calcium and, hence, in vegetable and animal tissue as a trace contaminant of calcium. The relative amount is, however, normally small, about one part per thousand of calcium, so that delicate methods of assay were required. Harrison (10) adapted the new technique of neutron activation analysis to this purpose, though latterly flame spectrophotometry has been utilized to give increased output (11).

Other laboratories (12, 13) have also been investigating the human metabolism of strontium, administering radioactive strontium, usually strontium 85, to subjects in the terminal stages of certain incurable diseases; there is naturally a certain hesitancy to give radioactive materials to subjects with a normal expectation of life and especially to children, except in very small doses. While one may justifiably be somewhat dubious of the validity of metabolic data obtained from subjects in cachectic states just prior to death, in fact the results of tracer studies obtained in this way agree very closely with those obtained from our normal volunteers given stable strontium in much larger amounts when measured as mass.

The metabolism of strontium must be considered in parallel with that of its chemical analogue calcium. It has even become fashionable to consider the two together and to record ratios. However it is imperative to remember that calcium is an essential mineral whereas stable strontium, while universally associated with calcium, is generally considered to be a casual trace-element, though some claim for it an essential role in ossification (14). Moreover, the relative concentrations differ by a thousandfold more or less, and this must be of importance when physical phenomena like solution and diffusion are involved. It is meet, therefore, to summarize what is believed to be the story of calcium metabolism, though the whole story is yet far from being understood.

Calcium Metabolism

In radiobiological jargon, we talk about the standard man (15). This hypothetical creature is not the statistically average man; he is more an ideal. As yet, unfortunately, he has no standard female counterpart and no standard children. This representative adult contains in his body rather more than a kilogram of calcium, of which all but about 1 gram will be in the skeleton.

The one gram or so in the soft tissues is mainly in solution in the blood plasma and the saline solution that diffuses out of the vascular system into the extracellular water. Its concentration is maintained within narrow limits in the physiological state, as is that of potassium, the balance between the two determining the normal degree of irritability of protoplasm.

Calcium and, presumably, strontium are largely but not completely excluded from the interior of the cells so that the concentration is higher in extracellular than intracellular water. Within the cell, and particularly within the nucleus, these cations play a part in binding nuclear proteins (16).

In blood plasma some of the calcium is bound loosely and reversibly to protein, chiefly albumin (cf. Fig. 29).

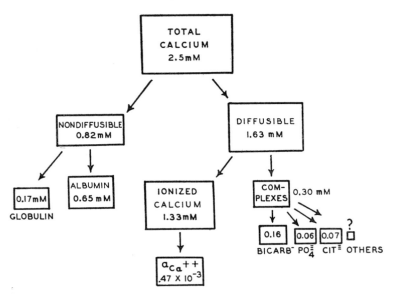

Fig. 29.—The state of calcium in normal serum as calculated from ultrafiltration data and formation constants. In ignoring possible ion competition—with Mg^{++}, for example—the amount of calcium estimated to be complexed may be in error (too high). This error could hardly affect the estimated ionized calcium by more than 2 or 3 per cent, however. mM designates mM/l. (From W. F. Neuman and M. W. Neuman, *The Chemical Dynamics of Bone Mineral* [Chicago, 1958], Fig. I-5.)

$$Ca^{++} + Protein \rightleftharpoons Ca\ Proteinate$$

Therefore calcium is mainly in the ionic form (about $\frac{2}{3}$ of the total) but a small amount, of the order of 1 per cent, is complexed with citrate and similar organic acids. It is only the ionic and soluble complexed calcium which can diffuse into extracellular water. Phosphate ions are also present in plasma and extracellular water, and it is notable that the concentrations of calcium and phosphate ions are such that the solution is supersaturated.

The greater than 99 per cent fraction of calcium in the body is in the skeleton, of which the mineral phase is composed mainly of hydrated calcium phosphate (apatite) crystals. About one-quarter of the skeleton is water, one-quarter organic matter, and one-half mineral. Part of the skeleton is of dense ivory bone like the shafts of the long bones, and part a spongework of trabeculae or little plates, as in the vertebrae and ends of the long bones.

Although growth in the exact sense of the term, enlargement, has ceased by the time the adult state is reached, bone is still in a dynamic state. Apposition of new bone and erosion of old bone are in continual process, but the two balance to give the steady state. The new bone must come from material supplied by the plasma and extracellular water, supersaturated in calcium phosphate. The eroded salts must be removed, paradoxically, by the same supersaturated vehicle.

Thus, while the bony skeleton can be considered in theory as a body compartment of constant size receiving from the extracellular fluid a steady contribution and giving up a similar amount to maintain the status quo, the plasma and extracellular water can be considered as another hypothetical compartment of constant size exchanging with the bone compartment and also receiving from the diet via the gut a steady flow of calcium and phosphate and giving up to the excreta a corresponding amount to maintain constancy (Fig. 30).

It is probable that the constancy of the fluid compartment is the vital factor. If the concentration of calcium ion falls, the unduly high irritability of protoplasm from the unbalanced action of potassium leads to the condition of tetany. If the concentration rises too far, the heart muscle may fail due to inadequate contraction. The bone compartment acts as an enormous reservoir of calcium which can discharge to the fluid compartment when the need arises and can be recharged when the critical period is over.

In fact at any point in time, the skeletal reservoir is nothing like so large as the figures suggest, some 1,000 times greater a mass of

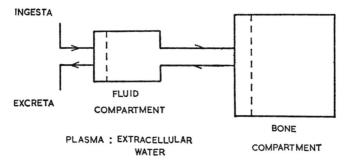

INGESTA

EXCRETA

FLUID
COMPARTMENT

PLASMA : EXTRACELLULAR
WATER

BONE

COMPARTMENT

EXCHANGEABLE : NON-EXCHANGEABLE
BONE   BONE

Fig. 30.—Simple model of "compartments" of the body into which
calcium and strontium are distributed.

calcium than that of the fluid pool. If one injects experimentally
a small dose of radioactive calcium intravenously into the fluid
compartment, this equilibrates over the course of a few minutes
with the whole of the extracellular pool and, apart from the fraction
excreted, within a few days with the "exchangeable" part of the
bony compartment. Bauer and his colleagues (17) calculated from
their experiments that the total exchangeable pool in man was
about 5 grams of calcium, that is about 1.5 grams in the fluid pool
plus 3.5 grams in the bone pool.

The exchange process is largely the physicochemical process of
ion exchange at the surface of bone crystals. The process can be
followed in vitro by placing powdered bone crystals into solutions
containing radioactive Ca^{45}

$Ca\ Phos + Ca^{45++} + Phos^=$

$$= Ca\ Phos + Ca^{45}\ Phos + Ca^{45++} + Ca^{++} + Phos^=.$$

The radioactive Ca ions in solution enter the bone surface to re-
place stable Ca ions which leave it. The activity of the solution
falls and that of the bone powder rises until ultimately a state of
equilibrium is reached. This process of ion exchange in bone both
in vitro and in vivo has been the subject of considerable research,
much of which has been carried out and summarized by Neuman

and his co-workers (18) in Rochester, N.Y. The picture given in its simplest form above is considerably more complex than this. There are at least three parts to the process (Fig. 31), the entry of the marked atom into the hydration shell covering the crystal surface, the exchange with atoms on the crystal surface, and exchange between atoms on the surface and those deeper down, intracrystalline exchange.

Ions of many different kinds can be exchanged from solution onto the crystal surface. These may be basic, such as sodium, lead, or magnesium, on the one hand, or acidic, such as fluoride or bicarbonate on the other. This allows bone to be quite a substantial

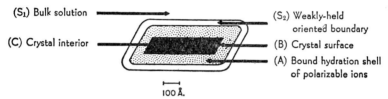

(S₁) Bulk solution

(C) Crystal interior

(S₂) Weakly-held oriented boundary

(B) Crystal surface

(A) Bound hydration shell of polarizable ions

100 Å.

Fig. 31.—A diagrammatic representation of a cross-section view of hydroxy-apatite crystal in aqueous suspension. (From W. F. Neuman and M. W. Neuman, *The Chemical Dynamics of Bone Mineral* [Chicago, 1958], Fig. IV-3.)

reservoir for ions other than calcium and phosphate and to be a buffer or sponge for mopping up certain excesses of useful or deleterious elements when the occasion warrants.

Most of this so-called heterionic, which I should prefer on etymological grounds to call allelionic, exchange is confined to the surface of the crystal. On physicochemical grounds it is possible for only a limited number of ions to enter the crystal lattice. Within the crystal, strontium and radium can substitute for calcium, and fluoride for the hydroxyl radical.

Thus the amount of exchangeable bone can be very appropriately measured by allelionic exchange with, say, radioactive sodium, Na^{24}. When radioactive calcium or strontium is used, there are two main processes operative, ion exchange and true bone formation with crystallization of apatite. However, by suitable handling of the experimental data, one can derive, as did Bauer *et al.* (17), the size of the total exchangeable pool and the daily internal loss from the pool in the formation of new bone. In these experiments on human subjects, the figure calculated was 0.5 gram per day of calcium passing from the total exchangeable pool of 5 grams of calcium into new bone.

One does not need all the trappings of modern technology, including radioactive tracers, to demonstrate the dynamic state of the bone. The microscope in the hands of histologists of former generations had revealed that new bone was being laid down by osteoblasts in foci in both ivory and, particularly, in trabecular bone and that old bone was being resorbed, the resorptive foci being characterized by giant cells called osteoclasts. Active areas often show part apposition and part resorption side by side. What can be shown by the radioactive tracer technique, for example marking the plasma-extracellular-fluid pool with an intravenous dose of Ca^{45}, is the pattern of transfer of these marked atoms to the bone. An injected animal's bones can be sampled by biopsy at intervals after giving the dose, or individuals from a group of identically managed animals can be sacrificed in series to give a time-course of events. The location of the radioactive atoms can be determined by radioautography. By this technique it can be shown that there are "hot spots" in the bone with a high concentration of the radioactive tracer, with rather variable concentrations elsewhere. The "hot spots" coincide with the areas which can be simultaneously visualized histologically as the foci of apposition.

What can be shown by another technique, microradiography (19) of thin plates of ivory bone, is that the units of this apparently uniformly dense bone are not equally opaque to these X-rays; that is, the concentration of mineral calcium varies. Sites of complete erosion can be identified; associated with them are areas of least density where early apposition is occurring, the hot spots of radioautography; and between these areas and the units of maximum density are others with various degrees of intermediate density.

It can be deduced, therefore, that units or areas of bone become activated in series. Erosion occurs, followed by nearby apposition.

Probably it is the sum of these active areas which make up the 3–4 grams of exchangeable bone at any one time. As one hole is filling up with new crystallization, another one forms.

The recently completed building site is formed of crystals of extremely small size, that is with a very large surface:volume ratio. Neuman (18) suggests that, while this is the perfect situation for ion exchange at the surface, the rushed job of construction has left many faults in the crystal which have to be made good later with intracrystalline exchange. This is a considerably slower process than surface exchange. It may be too that in vivo as in vitro crystal growth occurs, so that the final product is fewer crystals of larger size, greater perfection, and much less surface than the multitude of crystals first formed.

These physicochemical considerations of the maturation of bone units would be in accord with the microradiographic observations of a progressive increase in density of units up to a final maximum.

Formerly, bone physiologists and pathologists used to talk of "halisteresis," a solution of bone mineral without loss of organic ground substance. At the time it was felt necessary to invoke this concept to explain certain pathological phenomena connected with bone. In recent years "halisteresis" has become a dirty word. Certainly there does not now seem a need to invoke solution of bone salt to explain the pathological features of these diseases of bone. It may be inappropriate to use the same word for loss of atoms from maturing building sites, but I do believe from study of data on strontium that some such process must operate (*vide infra*).

We have come to the concept of a cyclical activation of units of bone with erosion and reapposition. What has not been certain is whether the life of such a unit is fixed within narrow limits, as for example is the life of the circulating red blood corpuscle of some 120 days in man; or whether the process is random in the statistical sense, that is that the life is determined by chance, some units having a short life, others a long life, but perhaps like radioactive nucleides with certain probabilities which lead to a determinable half-life. My own view is that not all bones are the same in structure. I have identified the broad distinction of ivory and trabecular bone, and there are probably nice distinctions within these broad limits. Depending on blood supply, function, and other factors, the life of the units is likely to vary. Again some evidence for this derived from data on strontium will be given (*vide infra*).

DEDUCTIONS FROM RADIOACTIVE CALCIUM

When a tracer quantity of radioactive calcium has been injected, as in the aforementioned experiments of Bauer, its concentration in plasma falls progressively with time (Fig. 32). When the con-

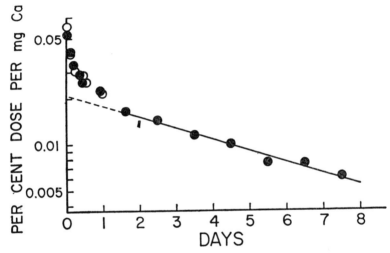

FIG. 32.—Specific activity of serum and urine Ca in one of the subjects plotted on a logarithmic scale against time. Symbols: ○ serum values; ● urine values. (From G. C. H. Bauer, A. Carlsson, and B. Lindquist, in Acta med. scand., **158**: 143, Fig. 1.)

centration is plotted against time, the form of the graph is curvilinear: even when the logarithm of the concentration is plotted against time, the graph is still curvilinear, though it is possible to postulate that this feature is the sum of a number of linear components each showing a less steep slope than its predecessor. This would be compatible with the marker's dilution in successive compartments. Uniform mixing in the blood plasma itself should be complete in a matter of minutes: simultaneously what was not protein-bound in the plasma would diffuse into the much larger extracellular space, and uniform mixing there should be complete within the hour; other probable processes are exchange to some extent with intracellular contents and ion exchange with the atoms on the surfaces of bone crystals (exchangeable bone). Excretion would be going on throughout.

In an experiment in which the concentration of activity in plasma can be measured or inferred for about 10 days, as in Bauer's cases, the terminal part of the log-linear graph appears to be a straight line. It has been customary to regard this part of the graph as indicative of the rate of loss of material from the exchangeable space by incorporation into bone plus loss by excretion. Since the excretion is measured, the bone-formation rate is calculated by difference.

The argument quoted from Bauer *et al.* (20) from experiments in which the uptake by the midshaft of tibias of young rats was measured is as follows:

This observation may be expressed mathematically as follows:

$$B_t^* = k_1 S_t^* + k_2 \int_O^t S^*(t) \, dt \qquad (1)^1$$

where B_t^* is the amount of isotope in tissue B at time t; S_t^* is the specific activity of the element (i.e. activity per unit weight of the element) in serum at time t; $\int_O^t S^*(t) \, dt$ is the area under the specific activity curve of the element in serum between time O and time t, and k_1 and k_2 are constants. . . .

The authors then made a case that the mathematical constants k_1 and k_2 can be equated to biological functions:

. . . one can rewrite Eq. (1) as follows:

$$B_t^* = E S_t^* + A \int_O^t S^*(t) \, dt \qquad (2)$$

[1] The expression

$$\int_O^t S^*(t) \, dt$$

for the integrated serum specific activity is identical with the expression $T \times S_M$ . . . in which S_M is the mean serum specific activity up to T time units following isotope administration. The present notation has been chosen to conform with common usage.

where E is the amount of exchangeable element in bone and A is the rate of accretion of the element; i.e. rate of incorporation into the nonexchangeable fraction of the bone salt.

. . . .

Based on Eq. (2) A and E may be calculated according to several alternative methods, giving slightly differing results. For example, Bauer *et al.* (1957a [17]) and Bauer and Ray (1958 [21]) used the following approach.

If the *minimum* lifespan (not to be confused with average lifespan) of the bone salt is longer than the length of time required for equilibrium of labeled calcium within the exchangeable calcium E, an exponential decrease in the activity of the exchangeable calcium, E_t^*, will be observed, once equilibrium has been attained, since $dE_t^* = -k'E$, where k' is the fractional removal rate. Plotted against time, the logarithm of the activity and of the specific activity of the exchangeable calcium will therefore appear as a straight line. The half-time, $T_{1/2}$, of this exponential will equal ᵗᵚe fractional removal rate from E,

$$k' = 0.693/T_{1/2}. \tag{3}$$

If accretion and excretion remove, from E, a and u units/time unit, respectively, of a material at specific activity S_t^*, and if 1 unit of activity was administered at zero time, then, at any interval until labeled material starts to return from the nonexchangeable fraction,

$$1 = E_t^* + (a + u) \int_O^t S^*(t) \, dt. \tag{4}$$

At activity equilibrium

$$E_t^* = ES^* \tag{5}$$

and since

$$k'E = a + u \tag{6}$$

substitution in Eq. (4), division of all terms by E, and inversion gives

$$E = 1/(S_t^* + k' \int_O^t S^*[t] \, dt). \tag{7}$$

Equation (7) can be solved for E by experimental determination of S_t^*. Equation (6) can then be solved for $(a + u)$, and as u can be experimentally determined $\left(u \int_O^t S^*[t] \, dt = \text{excretion} \right)$ a will be obtained.

It was in this way that these authors arrived at values for the exchangeable calcium in the body and the rate of accretion (or, I should prefer, apposition) of calcium to bone (but *vide infra*).

Formerly, no such direct method of estimating rates of bone formation was available. Instead indirect methods based on metabolic balance of intake versus output had to be considered. This procedure is still of value, especially in clinical medicine in pathological as well as physiological states.

CALCIUM BALANCE

The intake of calcium per day in the average adult of the United Kingdom is about 1.2 gm. according to the statistics of the Ministry of Agriculture, Fisheries and Food (22). About two-thirds of this calcium is provided by milk and milk products. In other countries, especially the oriental, the dietary calcium is provided mainly by vegetable sources, particularly cereals which have a high phosphate:calcium ratio. Much of the phosphate is due to phytic acid.

The problem is, therefore, "Are the phosphates, phytates, etc., which are sparingly soluble or almost insoluble in water, as available a source of calcium as milk?" In the latter, most of the calcium is only loosely bound to protein, so that on digestion in the intestinal tract calcium is, presumably, freed and becomes ionic.

During World War II, in order to preserve all the nutrients of the grain and because of the shortage of food supplies, the degree of extraction of flour was progressively raised in the United Kingdom, so that an increasing amount of phytate was retained. To counter this, flour was fortified with mineral chalk, which after contact with the hydrochloric acid in the stomach should be converted to chloride and ionized. Although the wartime high extraction of flour is now no longer practiced, fortification with chalk still remains.

The value of fortification was examined by McCance (23) studying the balances of individuals. The daily diet is standardized and the calcium intake measured. All excreta, urine and feces, are collected and measured separately for calcium. In the perfect steady state

intake = output (urine + feces).

Other sources of loss, such as from the skin by sweating and desquamation, are usually neglected, though some consider this loss to be quite considerable. What is excreted in the urine has certainly been absorbed and passed through the body; what is discharged in the feces is compounded of the true excretion from the body to the bowel, the endogenous fraction, and the rejection of unabsorbed calcium, the exogeneous fraction. Thus, while the parameters one would like are

$$A_b = \text{the calcium absorbed}$$
$$U = \text{the urinary calcium}$$
$$F_{en} = \text{the endogenous fecal calcium,}$$

so that one could compare A_b with $U + F_{en}$, in practice one cannot determine either A_b or F_{en} without the aid of something like radioactive markers. An approximation has to be made:

A_b' (apparent absorption) $= I$ (intake) $- F$ (total feces).

In the steady state $A_b' = U$. When $A_b' < U$ or $A_b' > U$, a negative or positive balance respectively is deduced.

Balance studies on the physiological adult in the steady state might show—intake-1.2 gm.:urine-0.3 gm.:feces ∼0.9 gm. per day. Here if A_b' ($= 0.3$ gm/day), the apparent daily absorbed calcium, mixed uniformly with all the body calcium of 1,050 gm., the average time for turnover of the body calcium would be

$$1{,}050 \times \tfrac{1.0}{3} \text{ day} = 3{,}500 \text{ days } (\sim 10 \text{ years}).$$

In fact studies with radioactive tracers such as Ca[45] show that the real absorption is greater than the apparent absorption; that endogenous fecal excretion is about half the urinary excretion of calcium, and, as we have noted, the absorbed calcium mixes uniformly with only a small fraction, rather than the whole, of the total body calcium, at least in the short term. Indeed about half the absorbed marker is excreted within a week or so. Thus, while A_b, the true daily absorbed calcium from the diet, might well be as much as 0.5 gm., the net amount available for bone formation is less than 0.3 gm/day.

It is important to stress at this stage that the body makes a considerable effort to preserve calcium. Excretion by the kidney involves a filtration of the diffusable fraction of the plasma (with a calcium concentration of about 67 mg/1) by the glomeruli at a rate of about 7 liters/hour (0.4–0.5 gm. Ca filtered per hour) and reabsorption by the tubules of all but a few per cent (an average of 12.5 mg/hour if the daily urinary excretion is 0.3 gm/day). It has been suggested (24) that all the ionic calcium is reabsorbed and that what escapes to urine is the diffusible but unionized, complexed calcium. A similar process operates in the gut. The gut contents consist not only of food but secretions from the salivary glands downward, all of which contain salts, including those of calcium. This addition to dietary calcium may reasonably be estimated (25) as 0.5–1 gm. a day; but, as tracer studies indicate that little over 100 mg. of endogenous calcium is lost in the feces daily, presumably this calcium must be more readily absorbed again than dietary calcium. The principle is clear; once calcium is absorbed, the body makes vigorous efforts to retain it by recycling both in kidney and gut.

Therefore, with the absorbed dietary calcium plus the recycled calcium to maintain the levels in the fluid pool, the amount of calcium converted into bone daily could in fact be quite large. The greater the recycling that occurs between bone compartments and fluid compartments, the greater could be the absolute rate of calcification of bone. Looking at the problem another way, we can say of the calcium atom absorbed from the diet that, though it has a high probability of relatively early excretion, once it gets incorporated into bone its chance of getting out of the body is low, though it does not necessarily stay in the same bone unit.

Balance studies, which form a large part of the foregoing argument, are not only inherently approximations, they are also difficult to carry out and very consuming of time and labor. To smooth out errors they should be conducted over substantial periods of time, which makes them still more expensive in effort. One can therefore always criticize them on the grounds of too short a coverage in time. This is important too since the mechanisms in the body for insuring homeostasis of calcium seem to be but crudely adjusted. Adaptation to changed intake is alleged to be slow, and one criticism (26) of the balance studies of McCance, which indicated a lower availability of calcium with a diet of high-extraction flour, has been that the period of study was too short. The critics claim that with longer periods adaptation does occur; possibly an enzyme, phytase, is built up in the adaptive process to free the calcium from this bound form and ultimately make it available for absorption. Certainly, unless cereal and vegetable calcium is available, it is difficult to see how people living on vegetable diets low in calcium (0.2–0.3 gm/day) can maintain healthy bones as they appear to do.

On diets low in calcium like the above, the excretion of calcium in the urine is low, perhaps only one-third of that for the representative adult of the United Kingdom. Correspondingly, the fraction of the dietary calcium apparently absorbed, according to balance studies, is high. The absolute amount absorbed appears to vary with the logarithm of the amount in diet.

Provided the content of vitamin D in the diet is adequate, calcium is absorbed according to the body's need. Deficiency of vitamin D leads to imperfect absorption, the product of calcium and phosphate in plasma falls, and bones do not calcify properly; they show microscopically broad instead of the normal narrow bands of uncalcified organic matrix.

Defective absorption of calcium seems to be only part of the story, for if vitamin D is adequate and calcium only lacking in the diet, the microscopical appearance is not that of the above (osteomalacia) but of a diminished mass of normal bone (osteoporosis). This condition is seen in domestic animals, such as sheep grazed on pastures where the soil is deficient in calcium (27). The osteoporosis tends to be cyclical in the ewe: marked after lactation, with its physiological drain of calcium, and checked when the lamb is weaned. The bones earliest affected are the cancellous bones, which must have the most labile stores. Probably the same syndrome occurs in the human species when diets are inadequate in calcium alone. However, deficiencies of both calcium and vitamin D can occur together, causing confused pathological pictures.

In contrast to this physiological osteoporosis, there appear to be pathological osteoporotic states where the calcium drain is not excessive and yet the homeostatic mechanisms of the body do not seem able to adapt to a normal drain. A persistent negative calcium balance is thus manifest, which may be corrected by raising the dietary levels of calcium (28, 29).

At the present time our understanding of homeostasis is very incomplete. Maintenance of the normal levels of plasma calcium to balance potassium seems to be the prime requirement, and the skeleton provides the reserve. Probably the whole system of endocrine glands influences the skeleton, and disorders of this system affect the skeleton.

Most potent among these glands is the parathyroid. Overactivity of the gland leads to exaggerated transfer of calcium salts from bone to plasma and, simultaneously, to decreased reabsorption of phosphate by the renal tubules, presumably to maintain constancy of the product of calcium and phosphate in plasma. It also influences absorption of calcium from the gut. It is presumably the degree of activity of this gland which sets the control for day-to-day activity of the resorptive mechanism in bone with its associated osteoclasts. Pathological overactivity leads to another characteristic demineralization—*osteitis fibrosa.*

Prolonged overactivity of the thyroid, which results in general metabolic stimulation, also results in a state of osteoporosis. Hormones of the adrenal cortex have a depressant action on the cells of connective tissue of which bone is a specialized variety. And the pituitary gland, which influences all the other members of the endocrine set, has a growth hormone which has been shown to affect the calcium status.

Metabolism of Strontium

STABLE STRONTIUM IN DIET

It has already been noted that strontium occurs in natural sources along with calcium. Food comes from the soil either directly via plants or indirectly via animals that subsist on vegetation. Thus, if the strontium content of soil varies from place to place, foodstuffs may be expected to vary in content of strontium. This undoubtedly applies from country to country and even within a country. In the United Kingdom, for example, there are certainly focal areas of sufficiently high strontium concentrations to be workable as commercial sources of strontium, including Strontian in Scotland from which the element got its name.

However, in the twentieth century in countries of advanced civilization like Great Britain, very few people live off their local land. Foods are imported and local products receive wide distribution within the country. Thus it is fair to take samples of food representative of the large supplies to the national larder, analyze them for strontium, sum the contributions according to national statistics of consumption, and obtain a mean figure for the representative diet. This is what my colleagues of the Agricultural Research Council's Radiobiological Laboratory (30) have done. They have analyzed samples of all the major sources of calcium in the national food for strontium and have derived a figure of 1.3 mg. of strontium per gram of calcium for the national diet or about 1.6 mg. per day for the representative diet with 1.2 gm. calcium. Naturally not every possible source of food has been analyzed; in fact, as noted, only those contributing substantially in calcium. It may be that certain foods contain significant quantities of strontium but little calcium, though this was considered unlikely.

Harrison (9, 31) in my own laboratory has conducted a small number of balance studies on members of our staff and their families, analyzing the composite diet for a period and comparing this with the output in urine and feces. For these few the daily intake has been somewhat higher than our colleagues' estimates: about 2–3 mg. per day for adults. We propose to analyze for strontium items of diets for which data are not yet available, for example sugar, where strontium preparations may be used in commercial processing.

ABSORPTION OF STRONTIUM

To measure this Harrison (9) first determined the daily output of natural strontium for several subjects, which as noted above was 2–3 mg. per day. They were then given a draught of 100–200 mg. of strontium as a soluble salt in water. The output naturally increased over the previous base line and was measurably in excess of this for about a month, by the end of which time about 20 per cent of the dose had been recovered in urine and 65 per cent in feces, leaving by difference some 15 per cent still retained, presumably in bone.

These figures indicate that some 35 per cent had been absorbed. Studies in other laboratories (13) with tracer doses of radioactive strontium give rather lower figures, around 20 per cent. The difference may well be due to a mass effect giving greater fractional absorption with the large doses. It is worthwhile recalling that qualitatively similar data have been obtained for calcium, but we have not studied the quantitative relations for strontium in man. Certainly around 20 per cent seems to be a fairly representative figure to take for absorption of soluble strontium salts.

The same considerations apply for strontium as previously considered for calcium—namely, are all dietary sources of strontium equally available? Whereas in the British diet some two-thirds of the calcium of the diet comes from dairy products and about 20 per cent from chalk, all of which may be in ionic form in the absorptive area of the gut, dairy products are relative to vegetable sources low in natural strontium (about 300 μg. per gram of calcium). Thus I (32) have calculated that of my own diet, containing a total of 2 mg. per day over a balance period, only about one-eighth came from dairy products, about three-eighths was derived from chalk (about 2.5 mg. per gram of calcium), and one-half from other sources, vegetable and unidentified. With the figures used in the calculation, it appeared that the strontium assumed to be of vegetable origin was considerably less well utilized than the remainder, though it was noted that any error in the assumptions would make a great difference in the answer obtained. Thus an experimental check is at present in progress. A number of subjects are living for several weeks on diets based on whole-meal bread, unfortified with chalk and obtained from grain grown on soil enriched with strontium 90, and milk from cows injected with strontium 85. Thus the cereal strontium will be marked with strontium 90, and the dairy strontium with strontium 85. The current and very incomplete results suggest that the former calculation was unreliable.

If in fact there is no great difference in availability of strontium and calcium depending on the dietary source, an apparent uptake of some 20 per cent of dietary strontium and of 40 per cent or more of dietary calcium, which Harrison (9) found in a balance period for which I was subject, would suggest that the mucosa of the intestinal tract is capable of some differentiation between the two ions. This has been confirmed by several laboratories (12, 13) using double-tracer techniques with radioactive isotopes of calcium and strontium in the diet of hospital patients and of normal experimental animals (33). It seems a general law applicable to mammals. It is not a general biological law. Roots of plants do not discriminate in uptake of calcium and strontium from culture solutions or normal soil water (34). Thus vegetable foodstuffs tend to have much the same ratio as the soils on which they are grown. Even within mammals it is apparently only certain physiological barriers which discriminate.

How strontium and calcium are absorbed from the gut is still a matter of considerable debate, as indeed is the whole subject of intestinal absorption. What appears certain is that it is only the small intestine which absorbs these ions; the rate is greatest in the uppermost part of this long tract, though the greatest mass may be absorbed lower down where the rate of flow is much slower (35).

Whether the absorption is a matter of simple diffusion down a concentration-gradient or whether work has to be done to transmit the ions across the mucosa or whether both processes operate is still undecided and so, therefore, is the process of discrimination. Studies (36) on isolated sacs of intestine removed from the body suggest that an active process involving expenditure of energy operates with calcium. Chemical agents which interrupt the cellular processes of energy-transfer inhibit the transport of calcium (37). It is of interest to note that Vitamin D facilitates the active transport of calcium in these experimental circumstances. Active transport of strontium has not been shown unequivocally with these systems. On the other hand, experiments, in which saline solutions were run through loops of gut into an intact blood supply in the living animal, have been interpreted (38) as supporting uptake by passive diffusion for strontium and for low concentrations of calcium.

EXCRETION OF STRONTIUM

Although it would be logical to consider the distribution of strontium once it has been absorbed into the plasma, there is some point in delaying this discussion, as will become apparent later, until excretion has been described.

As far as we are aware, the routes by which strontium is lost from the body are the same as for calcium. Whatever the process of absorption may be, only some 20 per cent of a single dose of radioactively marked strontium is absorbed, and the rest is discharged in the feces as exogenous fecal discard. As might be expected there is considerable variation between individuals. With a tracer dose given in this way by mouth, it is not possible to distinguish the unabsorbed discard from the true endogenous excretion, though one suspects that the exogenous material will have been largely cleared in a few days, the time again depending on the individual; but when the bulk is cleared one is left with a trickle which might be remnants of the exogenous waste or diminishing endogenous excretion.

ENDOGENOUS FECAL EXCRETION

The differentiation is decided with experiments which bypass the intestine. Thus, when radioactive strontium is given directly into the plasma, any fecal excretion must represent the endogenous component. The experiments of our own laboratory with normal subjects (9, 39) and of others with hospital patients (13) indicate that over the period of observation, which may range up to a month or so, only about 10 per cent of the injected dose in the representative adult is collected from feces. There is naturally a delay of a day or so from the injection to the peak value for percentage daily loss and then a progressive decline. The excretion by this route is but one-fifth to one-tenth of that in the urine over the same time.

In this respect, strontium is handled in man like calcium, but the other members of the alkaline earth group, barium and radium, which have a larger atomic mass, are excreted more by the fecal route. So, too, are strontium and calcium in many mammals, notably, the ruminants. There is scope here for further comparative physiological studies which might help to explain mechanisms.

It has been noted that phosphates, phytates, etc., of the diet may bind the calcium and strontium provided by the diet. Sulphates such as magnesium sulphate (Epsom salts) and sodium sulphate (Glauber salts) have been given experimentally to animals dosed by mouth with radioactive strontium, and some impairment of uptake has been noted; but the action here could be dual, involving not only the fixation as sparely soluble strontium salt but also intestinal hurry or purgation from the pharmacological action of sulphate. Perhaps agents like these bind endogenously secreted material too, but I know of no evidence in this connection. Calculations suggest endogenous and exogenous streams may be divorced: some 10–20 per cent only of the calcium reckoned to be excreted into the intestine appears in the feces while about half of the exogenous calcium is rejected.

Fatty acids will help to bind calcium and strontium as soaps in the intestinal tract. Certainly in the pathological states of sprue and idiopathic steatorrhea, signs of calcium lack may occur in the individual, which may be failure of uptake from the diet or binding of secretions, or both. On the other hand diets high in fat in normal subjects are said not to affect calcium status of the body. Thus the disease process, which is still unelucidated, in the pathological states is probably the common cause of both the steatorrhea and the failure adequately to maintain calcium balance.

Other chemical agents which bind calcium and strontium, such as citrates, if given by mouth, increase the loss of calcium in feces (40).

URINARY EXCRETION

The main route of excretion of strontium is undoubtedly in the urine. Relative to the fecal route, urinary excretion of strontium is apparently even greater than with calcium. Thus the hospital patients of Spencer and her colleagues excreted an average 39 per cent of intravenously injected strontium 85 in the urine against 14 per cent in feces in a 12-day period, whereas calcium 45 injected at the same time was partitioned, 14 per cent in urine and 10 per cent in feces (41).

The preferential excretion of strontium by the kidney compared with calcium has been recognized for many years. It was noted by Harrison (9) in his experiments where stable strontium was given by mouth to normal subjects, and he and his colleagues (42) have seen it too in short-term experiments following ingestion of short-lived strontium 87^m. The ratios, clearance of Sr^{87m}: clearance of calcium vary with individuals from about 3 to 4.5. This discrimination by the body against strontium combines with the absorptive discrimination to give a total discrimination of some fourfold between body fluids such as plasma and the diet. Comar and his colleagues (33) use this "observed ratio"

$$\frac{\text{Sr/Ca in compartment studied (e.g., plasma, bone)}}{\text{Sr/Ca in diet}}$$

as a useful index of total discrimination and also derive factors—discrimination factors (DF)—which indicate numerically the weighted effect of each process in the total discrimination. Thus again in hospital patients they (12) deduce that discrimination in absorption is the more important contribution. Nevertheless, the renal effect is a useful supplement.

If we neglect the possibility of secretion of strontium by the tubules of the kidney, we can explain renal discrimination between strontium and calcium as a preferential reabsorption of calcium by the tubules from the glomerular ultrafiltrate of plasma. Thus the discrimination exercised by the renal tubules could well be substantially similar to that of the intestinal mucous membrane.

Let it be remembered that the renal tubules reabsorb about 99 per cent of the calcium brought to them by the glomerular ultrafiltrate. Even with the observed preference for calcium, the degree of reabsorption of strontium from the ultrafiltrate is still about 98 per cent. Experimental studies by Chen and Neuman in dogs (24) suggest that, the major component of plasma-ultrifiltrate being ionic calcium and the minor one calcium complexed with citrate and similar radicals, the ionic calcium is reabsorbed and the complexed calcium discharged to the bladder. Possibly the same applies for strontium. If so, the ratio of complexed to ionic strontium in plasma should be higher than for calcium; but calcium is more readily complexed than strontium. However, as the source of citrate as a complexing agent is probably bone (see Neuman and Neuman [18, p. 142]), it may be that the efflux from bone to plasma has a high strontium:calcium ratio, though the influx from plasma to bone is generally accepted as without discrimination.

Leaving speculation aside we can look at the rate of urinary excretion of a marked dose of strontium. The various investigators, whether using radioactive tracers or stable strontium in doses of pharmacological size, agree that the maximum excretion is on the day of administration, be it oral or intravenous. Thereafter the percentage of dose excreted per day falls off progressively. When the logarithm of the daily urinary excretion is plotted against time, a curvilinear relationship is obtained. This can be expressed as the sum of a number of exponential processes

$$E_x = Ae^{-at} + Be^{-bt} + Ce^{-ct} \ldots,$$

Where E_x is the excretion per day at time, t and A, a, B, b, C, c, etc., are constants. The important thing as Harrison (9) and coworkers showed was that E_x, the urinary excretion rate, varied with the concentration in plasma (C_p)

$$E_x \propto Cp$$

or $$E_x = K\,Cp,$$

where K is constant and has the dimensions vol/time. Another way of saying this is that the volume of plasma cleared of strontium per unit time is constant. For a given individual under ordinary conditions of balance, this value is constant, whether the concentration we are considering is that of a radioactive tracer, like strontium 85 (Bishop *et al.* [39]), or an elevation of the natural stable strontium by a hundredfold or more (Harrison *et al.* [9]). Doubtless the value of this clearance may be changed by substantial restriction of diet or disturbed metabolism. Thus the clearance values for the normal subjects of our laboratory are:

G.E.H. = 0.44 ± 0.04 liter/hour
J.F.L. = 0.73 ± 0.07 liter/hour
R.H.M. = 0.50　　　liter/hour,

whereas data on hospital patients (Spencer *et al.* [41, Fig. 4]) on diets low in calcium (134 mg/day) varied from about 0.3 to 0.03. These patients had been under treatment for malignant disease or had diagnosis of bone disorder, notably osteoporosis, and these latter were in the lower end of the range quoted.

Practically all of the data obtained on excretion are from experiments in which a single dose of strontium has been given. Valuable though such information is for understanding the metabolism, these experiments have disadvantages. Intravenous injection inserts the whole dose into the plasma pool within a minute or so, which is not representative of the time scale of normal alimentary absorption. Oral doses of soluble salt may be representative, but this is not known, since the availability of various forms of strontium remains a question; in addition it seems from our experimental data (Barnes *et al.* [42]) that absorption may be quite different when strontium salts are given in solution on "an empty stomach" and after a meal (this is well known to physicians who give drugs before or after meals to take advantages of rapid or slow absorption). Since the time-course of entry of strontium into the circulation may affect its fate, one really requires information about multiple ingestions where the fluctuations would be smoothed out. From one short balance experiment for stable strontium in myself, the daily intake was 2 mg. and the urinary output 0.4 mg. or 20 per cent of the intake. This may well be representative for me as an individual, but it is likely to be a value at the upper end of the range of normal, since my output of both calcium and strontium is the highest recorded in our laboratory. Current experiments in which diets of a few of our staff are labeled should provide a better answer.

OTHER SOURCES OF LOSS

Skin, by desquamation and through sweating, has been cited as a source of loss of calcium. Values for sweat of 2–7 mg. per 100 ml. have been recorded (43). I am not aware of similar data for strontium, though unpublished observations of ours are that strontium 85 could but doubtfully be detected in clothing worn for 24 hours and in swabs from skin of subjects with readily measurable strontium 85 in their plasma. To neglect loss of strontium from the skin in balance studies thus seems justifiable.

The mammary glands are greatly modified sweat glands of considerable significance in mammals. Comar and his colleagues (44) have reported that in 4 out of 5 lactating women the concentration of strontium 90 relative to calcium was on average one-tenth of that in their diet and deduced that this indicated preferential secretion of calcium. This would be in accord with their observations of preferential secretion of calcium in other experimental mammals.

About this result, which has most important implications in favor of breast feeding, I still have some reservations and would welcome more data, since our unpublished observations, which are very few, indicate little difference between the ratios of stable strontium to calcium in plasma and milk of the same lactating women. It is well known that lactation causes a drain on the skeleton. Under these circumstances plasma may reflect specific activity of the bone rather than diet. Thus, while the observations are undoubtedly sound, the conclusion from them must be validated.

The placenta in the pregnant woman is a barrier between the maternal and fetal circulations. Comar's group (33) have led again in showing that discrimination between strontium and calcium occurs at this barrier in experimental animals. Once again calcium is passed preferentially to the fetus. The same applies in the human subject. From survey data Bryant (45) and his colleagues find the strontium:calcium ratio in the bones of stillborn infants in the United Kingdom to average 200 $\mu g/g$. The same analysts find adult bone to average 320 $\mu g/g$, which is much the same figure as Harrison (9) finds in plasma of adults. The discrimination factor in man may not be quite as great as the twofold found in other species, but it is substantial.

BLOOD-BONE RELATIONSHIPS

As in calcium metabolism, blood-bone relationships here are of greatest interest, since they are the foundation of our understanding of mineralization of bone. Since we are, in the case of strontium 90, interested in hazard from radiation dose, the blood-bone relation is of still greater interest.

The strontium, be it stable strontium, strontium 85, or strontium 90, enters the blood stream by absorption from the gut. We have seen how most of it, while it is the blood plasma, is recycled through the gut and through the kidney with some loss in each to feces and urine. In each case the percentage loss per cycle is small, but the aggregate is substantial.

Just as calcium 45 has been administered and followed to elucidate the blood-bone relationships of calcium, so also has strontium 85 been used for strontium. In many respects strontium 85 has advantages as has been pointed out: a low radiation dose to bone per microcurie administered and the emission of a γ-ray which allows it to be followed from without by whole-body counting.

Bauer with Ray (21) has reported his results of injecting strontium 85 intravenously into 5 essentially normal adult subjects and has analyzed the results obtained over the subsequent 5 days with the aid of an electronic analogue computer. From the exercise a model (Fig. 33a) was derived. The box B is taken as the plasma compartment of unit size which exchanges with compartments X and Y of sizes 6.4 and 3.0 with respect to B, and Y exchanges with another larger compartment of size 9.0. Excretion is reckoned to occur from the plasma compartment and apposition of new bone (accretion) from Y, which is interpreted as being the extracellular fluid compartment. The rates of exchange and loss from the compartments given in Figure 33b and the compartment sizes were derived from the computer's data. It is admitted that the cumula-

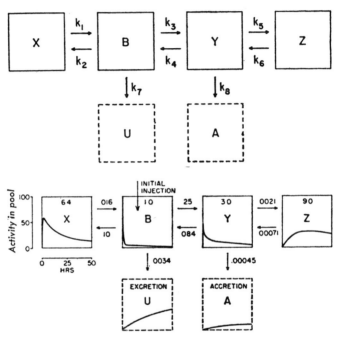

FIG. 33.—*3-A*: Drawing of postulated model for strontium metabolism. Compartment B represents the vascular space (serum). The nature of compartments X, Y, and Z is unknown. Excretion and accretion proceed at rates k_7 and k_8, respectively. The boxes U and A, containing activity drained from the system by excretion and accretion, have been outlined with dots to symbolize that they do not represent true compartments: uniform mixing is not presumed to occur in, for instance, the accretion box. *3-B*: Schematic drawing of the observed serum and excretory activity (B* and U*) simulated with an electronic analogue computer. The figures within the boxes indicate relative volumes derived from the k values, the volume of B being the unit of reference. (The rate constants k_1–k_8 are expressed in terms of decimal fractions per minute.) For comparison, the activity-time curves for the first 50 hours following administration of activity into B are schematically indicated. (From G. C. H. Bauer, and R. D. Ray, in *J. Bone & Joint Surg.*, 40: 171, Figs. 3-A and 3-B.)

tion of the curves for disappearance of strontium 85 from the blood and for its appearance in excreta was by trial and error, so that the model derived is not necessarily the only one. Compartment X is interpreted as intracellular fluid and Z as exchangeable bone.

My only criticism of this elegant work would be of the interpretation. It is difficult for me to envisage how any intracellular water (box X) other than that of the circulating blood cells can be in direct exchange with plasma. My picture is that the vast mass of intracellular water must exchange with extracellular water. Furthermore, I should not expect the volume of intracellular water to be so large, unless the cell membranes are unique in discriminating for strontium against calcium. If box X is not intracellular water, it is about the right size for exchangeable bone—a possibility which I infer Bauer and Ray do not exclude. In confirmation of this is its rapid equilibrium with plasma which would be expected of exchangeable bone in vivo, if studies with bone in vitro are any guide.

If box X is really exchangeable bone equilibrating with extracellular water, box Y, rather than directly with plasma, one still has to account for box Z. This might well be a further exchangeable part of bone perhaps slower intracrystalline exchange.

The important factors are, however, not the intermediate but the ultimates, accretion box A and excretion box U. The latter has a considerably higher rate than the former. Thus Figure 34, also from Bauer (20), indicates some 50 per cent excretion and 20 per cent "accretion" after 5 days, with 30 per cent still "exchangeable."

I am naturally more familiar with the details of experiments in my own laboratory (39), when both Harrison and I have received a single dose of 0.5 μc. of strontium 85 intravenously. We were able to follow the changes in concentration of strontium 85 in plasma by direct measurement for 2 days. We also have observations on the concentration in urine up to 90 days in one case and 150 days in the other. Although the stable strontium in plasma and urine was not measured in this experiment, we have previous observations. Since these values are roughly constant we can make approximations as to the specific activity of urine strontium 85/stable strontium. Since the urine should be of the same specific activity as the plasma from which it is derived, we can calculate the approximate concentration of strontium 85 in plasma for 90 and 150 days respectively. Figure 35 shows for myself as subject the strontium 85 free in extracellular water, calculated from the observed values in plasma/liter × 13.2, as a fraction of the total retained strontium 85, the latter being derived from observations on intake-excretion and on retention as determined by whole-body monitor.

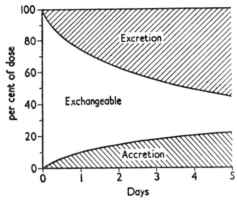

Fig. 34.—Distribution of strontium 85 following intravenous injection in man. The graph has been drawn on the basis of values obtained by Bauer and Ray (1958). In contrast to *rats*, even 5 days following administration as much as 50 per cent of the activity retained in *man* is still in the exchangeable fraction. (From G. C. H. Bauer, A. Carlsson, and B. Lindquist, in *Mineral Metabolism*, ed. C. L. Comar and F. Bronner, I [1961], Part B, 609, Fig. 12.)

Between 5 and 150 days this fraction of strontium 85 free in plasma can be expressed as the sum of two exponential processes. Up to 5 days this curve for plasma as for urine is the sum of several more rapid processes.

We have no data about concentrations after 150 days as the activity was too small to measure. However, a few observations are available on the change of concentration of strontium 90 in urine on subjects contaminated while at work with this isotope (46, 47). The rate of change of concentration in urine in these subjects altered at about 150 days and a still slower rate operated for the next 6 months or more.

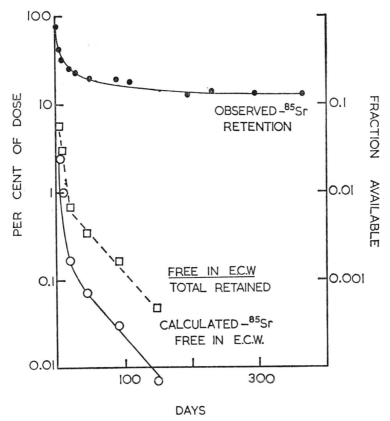

FIG. 35.—Strontium 85 in man after intravenous injection. Symbols: ●————●, Observed percentage retention of dose of Sr[85] (log scale—left hand ordinate) versus time; ○————○, Calculated percentage of a single dose of Sr[85] free in extracellular water (log scale —left hand ordinate) versus time; □————□, Calculated fraction of ○————○ / ●————● (log scale—right hand ordinate) versus time. (Data derived from Bishop *et al.*, in *Internat. J. Rad. Biol.*, **2:** 125.)

Provided the urinary excretion rate is always a constant function of plasma concentration, as the urinary excretion rate is continuously declining in rate, so too will plasma concentration be declining. The pattern, which was described under calcium metabolism, of a progressively declining rate at the beginning easing into a constant exponential rate is valid when the period of observation is limited, but, with the advantage of higher activities for injection and easier counting for γ-emitters, it can be shown that the period of constant rate is relatively short.

Bluhm *et al.* (48) using calcium 47 have shown that the same phenomenon may be observed with calcium isotopes, a break occurring after about 10 days.

It is meet to ask what all this means.

In the experiments of Bauer and his colleagues (17), described above, the reasonable and classical postulate was made that in the first day or two the changing rate of decline of the concentration of isotope in plasma was due to mixing in, that is exchange with the various compartments of soft tissue and with exchangeable calcium of the bone. By the end of this period, equilibrium had been established with the soft tissue, and the constant rate of decline from then till 10 days represented loss from the exchangeable pool to excreta and bone. Now it is certain that when calcium or strontium is excreted from the body it is irretrievably lost; but when it is taken up by bone, whether by exchange or by crystallization of bone salt, it can be brought back into circulation. Hence Bauer's emphasis (p. 100) that the minimum life span in bone salt had to be substantial if his equations were to be meaningful.

The change in rate of decline at about 10 days could be due to return of the marker from slowly equilibrating space into which "diffusion" (Bluhm *et al.* [48]) had taken place or from bone salt of a temporary nature as envisaged by Heaney and Whedon (49). This temporary bone could be a scaffolding rather than a permanent structure, that is "halisteresis" may be a normal process. Neuman (18) describes how, initially, crystallization is a rapid producing of small imperfect crystals of great surface area. Since these areas of primary crystallization must be relatively easily accessible to the circulating plasma, it is likely they represent not only primary crystallization but, in virtue of their crystal surfaces, the "readily exchangeable" bone too. Later these areas mature, crystals are perfected, grow in size, and there is a general increase in density.

Whether the bone-formation rate as calculated by Bauer includes a factor which is diffusion or formation of evanescent calcium bone salt is of academic importance only. The net bone formation is less than analysis of this particular exponential would suggest. The data derived from experimental administration of strontium 85 and accidental contamination with strontium 90 take the problem very much further than the 10 days or so of Bauer or the few weeks of Bluhm *et al.* and Heaney and Whedon. They indicate that more and more strontium is returning to the plasma from cyclical processes with a progressively longer average life. The plasma concentration (Ct) of marked strontium at any time t, like the urinary excretion rate, can be expressed as a series of exponential terms:

$$Ct = Ae^{-at} + Be^{-bt} + Ce^{-ct} + \ldots,$$

from which it could be interpreted that the strontium was extending into and equilibrating with successively larger spaces.

One process certainly is not reversible, excretion. However, from experimental data it is easy to correct for excreta; and elsewhere (32) I have calculated the total strontium 85 free in extracellular water versus time after injection and expressed it as a fraction of the retained strontium. From this, one can derive compartment sizes and rate constants. The approximate numbers were $A = 2.75$ mg., $B = 40$ mg. of natural strontium, $a = 0.14/\text{day}$, $b = 0.018/\text{day}$, for myself as subject, and, as a guess, $C > 150$ mg., and $c = 0.003/\text{day}$. If these numbers were meaningful, the first compartment would be near equilibrium with the exchangeable pool in a few weeks, the second in a few months, and the third, which would comprise a substantial fraction of the skeleton (300–400 mg. of strontium), in a few years.

However, I doubt if this relatively simple picture is realistic. Although as a model it is usual to consider the body as a series of compartments or fixed structures, the skeletal compartments would appear from histological and radioautographic evidence to be dynamic and changing.

We have the physiological and pathological evidence that can-cellous bone and certain cancellous bones in particular are more labile than ivory bone. For ivory bone, we have, it is true, the microradiographic evidence from Amprino and Engstrom (19) that at any particular time different units are of varying density, and therefore completeness of calcification, up to a maximum; but we do not know whether the renewal is random or selective. Radioautographs show "hot spots"—the foci of early ossification soon after injection of radioactive isotopes (50, 51) (Fig. 36), but later, although hot spots are still evident, the total activity per unit bone is diminishing and the dispersion of marker is considerable (52).

My conclusion is that, while all we can see of the mechanisms are wheels within wheels within wheels, developed in evolution, we cannot yet feed this information into our estimates of hazard of strontium 90. Instead we can take a much simpler and empirical attitude. From the experiments in which strontium 85 has been given to the human adult, we can say that about one-seventh of the injected material is still present in the skeleton at the end of a year. From the data on retention, we can see that the rate of loss from the body is then very slow. Stable strontium which follows the same pathway is taken in by the British subject at the rate of 2 mg. per day, and about 20 per cent is absorbed, of which one-seventh is due for slow turnover,

$$\tfrac{1}{7} \times \tfrac{1}{5} \times 2 \approx \frac{0.06 \text{ mg.}}{\text{day}}.$$

British bone contains about 0.05 mg. strontium per gram. Thus definitive bone formation is just over a gram a day, say 400 grams a year or some 6 per cent replacement per year. This is about 3 times less than Bauer's estimate based on an apposition rate of 0.5 g. of calcium a day, but this was, as we have seen, apposition of temporary as well as definitive bone. It may still be too high, as data derived from surveys of world-wide strontium 90 fallout may show.

Calcium and Strontium in Children

The understanding of the movement of strontium and calcium is difficult enough in the adult where a steady state operates. In

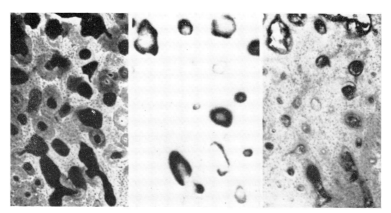

Fig. 36.—Microradiograph, autoradiograph, and photomicrograph of the same cross-section, from the shaft of the tibia of a young adult dog, killed 9 weeks after intravenous administration of strontium 90. Undecalcified, unstained, ground transverse section. × 62. (Prepared by Jenifer Jowsey. From F. McLean, in *Science*, **127**: 451. Reprinted from *Science* by permission.)

children there is the added complexity of growth. Furthermore, very little evidence is available from the modern techniques involving radioactive materials because of the natural reluctance of physicians to administer such substances to children. There is of course a substantial collection of older works on calcium metabolism of infants and children but very little on strontium. My colleagues have attempted to study children when opportunities are offered.

CALCIUM AND STRONTIUM IN DIET

The newborn infant is fed at the maternal breast or artificially, usually with cows' milk, neat or modified. Cows' milk having been produced for the much more rapidly growing calf has a high calcium content relative to human milk, rather more than a gram of calcium per liter compared with about one-quarter of a gram per liter of human milk. The concentration of stable strontium in British cows' milk is well documented, averaging about 0.4 mg. per liter. The few estimates we have been able to make on human milk give a strontium:calcium ratio little lower than cows' milk.

On the purely or largely milk diet, the infant doubles its birth weight in about 6 months and trebles it in a year. The amount of calcium in the body rises correspondingly. According to the data of Mitchell *et al.* (53) for children in the U.S.A., the calcium content at birth is about 30 grams and rises to about 100 at 1 year. This remarkable fractional rate growth is not maintained, though one sees on reference to Figure 37 that the absolute increase per year after the age of 1 year, while falling off for a few years, rises again to a peak around the years of puberty and then declines until the steady state is reached about the age of 20.

Depending on customs and circumstances the milk diet of the infant is supplemented with cereals and vegetables progressively in the first year. Subsequently he begins to eat a more varied diet. Statistics of British children (54)—rather out of date it is true—indicate, however, that the representative calcium intake is about 800 mg. of calcium a day at all ages in children. The strontium content of these diets was not analyzed, but it can be estimated

as rising progressively from about 0.5 mg/gm Ca in the first year
steadily up to the adult figure of perhaps 1.3–2 mg/gm Ca.

BALANCE STUDIES

In contrast to the normal adult in the steady state, who is in
exact balance in the long run—though over short periods such as
one can conveniently measure he might be in slight net loss or
gain—the infant and child are in considerable "positive" balance.
Infants on cows' milk, with its higher calcium content, show this
more strongly than breast-fed infants who, however, presumably
extract a higher proportion of the dietary calcium.

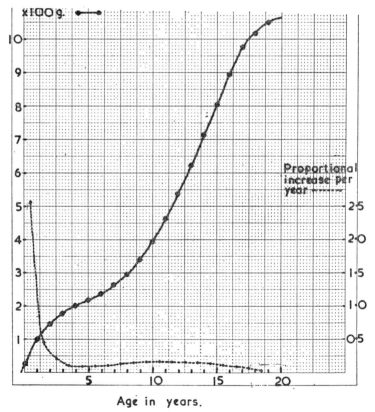

Age in years.

Fig. 37.—The mass of skeletal calcium (left hand ordinate) versus age,
and the proportional increase per year (right hand ordinate). (From data
derived from Mitchell, *et al.*, *J. Biol. Chem.*, **158**: 625.)

Very little information exists about natural strontium. My colleagues in conjunction with members of the Department of Experimental Medicine at Cambridge (55) have recorded balances of strontium and calcium for 3-day periods on infants a week old. The subjects were divided into two groups—the breast fed and the artificially fed. The calcium balances were as expected, both positive, and more strongly so in the artificially fed. The data for strontium, however, were a surprise. The artificially fed infants showed a net gain of strontium, while the breast fed showed a net loss of strontium during the 3-day period. Admittedly the period is a very short one, necessarily so because of technical and administrative difficulties, and it is not possible to say that the effect, which appeared real, is more than temporary. The authors explain the phenomenon thus. Breast milk has a much lower concentration of phosphate as well as calcium compared with cows' milk. The phosphate is an essential for the soft tissue metabolism and growth; think of the phosphate required for the nucleic acids, the keys to nuclear metabolism and protein synthesis. To insure an adequate supply of phosphate, the bones are burgled for their phosphate, and strontium and calcium are withdrawn with it. The calcium is preserved as far as possible by the natural mechanisms, but some strontium escapes in the excreta. This must mean that the excretory mechanisms, notably in the kidney which retains calcium in preference to strontium, are fully or well developed at birth, though in other respects the kidney is then very immature. As a test of their hypothesis these workers fed phosphate as a supplement to breast milk to a further group of infants; these infants showed a net gain of strontium.

This drain of strontium from the body probably does not last long. Indeed the observed loss might even be the shedding of an accumulation during the previous months of fetal life due to the cycles which operate then but not later, excretion into the amniotic fluid followed by the ingestion of this bath water. Anyway the measurements made by my colleagues in surveys of the bones of infants (methods of feeding unspecified) do not show any remarkably greater variation in the strontium concentration in the first few months of life than at birth (45).

The older infants and children on a diet containing about 5–6 grams of calcium a week excrete a smaller amount of calcium in the urine than would the adult on a similar diet. The urine of children up to the age of puberty usually contains between 50 and 100 mg. of calcium per day, say 0.5 gm. per week. The retained calcium may well be around 1 gm. per week. Once again data for stable strontium are very scanty, but the following figures observed by my colleagues (56) are perhaps representative for excretion:

TABLE 3

INDIVIDUAL AND SEX	AGE		URINARY EXCRETION			FECAL DISCHARGE		
	Years	Months	Sr (Mg.)	Ca (Gm.)	Sr/Ca$\times 10^3$	Sr (Mg.)	Ca (Gm.)	Sr/Ca$\times 10^3$
S.R.W. ♂.......	4	10	0.049	0.039	1.25	0.62	0.50	1.24
M.A.L. ♀.......	9	9	0.104	0.093	1.12	1.26	0.77	1.63
A.S.H. ♂.......	{ (i) 13	1	0.109	0.087	1.25	3.46	1.42	2.44
	{ (ii) 14	4	0.093	0.083	1.12	2.35	0.97	2.42
R.M. ♂........	14	6	0.293	0.199	1.46	2.99	1.25	2.39

The figures suggest that, as in the case of calcium, the concentration of strontium in urine is several times lower than in adults of our laboratory who excrete 0.15 to 0.4 mg. a day and that the change may occur about puberty. Doubtless some of the difference is accounted for by diet, but there may well be an additional metabolic factor.

I am not aware of any studies on the balance of strontium in children. The data above were from the control period of an experiment in which these children drank a solution containing 100 mg. of natural strontium. The accountancy of this dose was as follows:

TABLE 4

	EXCRETION—PERCENTAGE OF DOSE			RETENTION—PERCENTAGE OF DOSE
	Urine	Feces	Total	
4 children.....	3.0 ± 0.4	77.7 ± 1.9	80.7 ± 2.2	19.3 ± 2.2
3 adults.......	18.5 ± 1.4	66.8 ± 0.8	83.3 ± 2.0	16.7 ± 2.0

This suggests that the degree of absorption was not greater in children than adults; indeed from the larger proportion of the dose in feces one might conclude that absorption was less, but there is no information about endogenous fecal loss. The notable feature is the different partition of absorbed material between retention and urinary excretion, the ratio being about 6:1 for children against 1:1 for adults. We cannot calculate clearances, as strontium values for plasma were not obtained. One can but estimate that the renal clearance, standardized to body size, is not greatly different from the adult, but the clearance by bone is relatively high.

Deductions from Surveys of Strontium 90

The previous accounts have been based on data collected in the laboratory where the circumstances are planned. The alternative approach is the analysis of data derived from survey. Strontium 90 has been liberated into the atmosphere by the explosion of nuclear weapons. The amounts were small and probably below the range of measurement until the development and explosion of megaton devices beginning in 1954. As far as the biologist is concerned these were not planned experiments. In fact in the United Kingdom a serious attempt was not made until the latter end of 1955 to follow the progression of strontium 90 from the atmosphere into foodstuffs and so into human bone.

STRONTIUM AND STRONTIUM 90 IN DIET

Since 1958 the effort given to the program of monitoring for strontium 90 has been increased. Notably, the Agricultural Research Council (57) has become responsible for measurement of the degree of contamination of the foods which provide substantial amounts of calcium in national diet and the assessment therefrom of the concentration of strontium 90 in the total diet.

Since dairy products provide some two-thirds of the calcium in the national diet, a particularly careful survey has been mounted for milk. For administrative purposes England is divided into 10 regions, which, with Scotland and Northern Ireland, make up 12 zones. The milk of the zones is sampled at source according to a statistical plan which covers 20 per cent of the milk produced in the country. The survey is done in duplicate, so that, in effect, 40 per cent of the country's production is measured. Cheese, both home-produced and imported, is also sampled. Vegetable sources of calcium, as cereals and root and leaf vegetables, are assayed in a similar but less comprehensive fashion.

Drinking water derived from the three types of source, reservoirs, rivers, and wells, is also examined. Since the numbers of people supplied by each type of source is known, the average contribution to the total diet from water can be computed.

By addition of the respective fractions, the assessment of the degree of contamination of the average diet is derived for 1958, 6.1 $\mu\mu$c/gm Ca; for 1959, 9.3 $\mu\mu$c/gm Ca; and for 1960, 6.4 $\mu\mu$c/gm Ca (Table 5).

TABLE 5

SOURCE OF STRONTIUM 90	ESTIMATED STRONTIUM 90 INTAKE ($\mu\mu$C/DAY)		
	1958	1959	1960
Diet			
Milk, cream, cheese..............................	4.20	5.57	3.67
Root vegetables.................................	0.35	0.58	0.49
Leaf and other vegetables, fruit..................	0.54	0.88	0.52
Flour and cereals...............................	0.75	1.32	1.07
Eggs, meat, fish, etc...........................	0.32	0.55	0.37
Total.......................................	6.16	8.90	6.12
Drinking water.................................	0.23	0.43	0.36
Tea...	—	0.45	0.45
Air breathed..................................	0.16	0.30	—
Total daily intake.............................	6.55	10.08	6.93
Daily intake $\mu\mu$c/gm Ca......................	6.1	9.3	6.4

A more limited survey in 1957 by Bryant *et al.* (57) indicated a value of 5.5 $\mu\mu c$/gm Ca. Prior to that, measurements specific for the purpose of estimating levels in diet were not made. However, it is known that the rate of fallout of strontium 90 in the United Kingdom was practically constant from May, 1954, through April, 1958, (0.2–0.25 mc/km²/month) (59). On this basis I have taken approximations for levels in diet as 2, 4, and 5 $\mu\mu c$/gm Ca for 1954, 1955, and 1956.

The average diet, containing 1.084 gm. of calcium a day including 0.24 gm. of mineral calcium from chalk in the fortified flour, is derived from the national statistics of the Ministry of Agriculture, Fisheries and Food. There is evidence from these statistics that the diet is representative for the British adult. What are not available are up-to-date figures of what children eat at various ages. A careful analysis of children's diets was made in the years just before World War II by Widdowson (54), who, to insure reliability, selected children of intelligent and co-operative parents. This probably biased the information to the then upper social classes. For purposes of calculation, since these are the only available data, I have used them, assuming that, with the rise in standards of living in the last 20 years, the average child of today will be equivalent to the upper-class child then.

While strontium 90 was being measured radiochemically, the opportunity was taken to measure the stable strontium of the dietary constituents spectrometrically. It was from these measurements that the previously quoted figure of 1.3 mg. of strontium per gram of calcium was obtained for the national diet. My calculation from Widdowson, based on the analytical figures of the A.R.C. Radiobiological Laboratory, for children's diets are given in Figure 38. They show a steady rise from 0.5 mg/gm Ca for the age of 1 to 1 mg/gm Ca for teen-agers.

When the figures for strontium 90 and stable strontium are both available, the true specific activity ($\mu\mu c$ Sr[90]/mg Sr) of the whole diet and its constituents can be derived. This gives a considerable advantage over the specific activity in terms of calcium ($\mu\mu c$ Sr[90]/gm Ca), since many of the complexities of strontium-calcium

STABLE   STRONTIUM   IN   BONE   AND   DIET

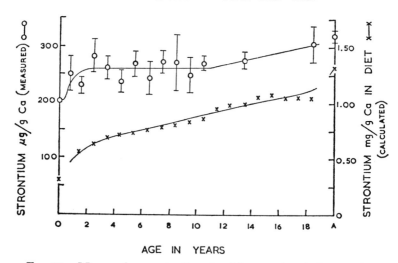

Fɪɢ. 38.—Measured concentration of stable strontium in bone and calculated concentration in diet according to age of United Kingdom subject
in years. From F. J. Bryant and J. F. Loutit, *Human Bone Metabolism
Deduced from Strontium Assays*, AERE–R 3718 (London, 1961).

discrimination are avoided. One is left only with the possibility of
selective absorption of strontium from different kinds of foods—
the problem of availability of dairy and vegetable strontium.

STRONTIUM 90 AND STRONTIUM IN BONE

   Contemporaneously with the increase in effort on monitoring
foodstuffs, Bryant of the Atomic Energy Authority has been able
to increase the number of samples of human bone analyzed for
strontium 90. In addition, another laboratory in Glasgow has
made a substantial number of measurements in 1959 and 1960.
   Unlike foods, human bones cannot be collected according to a
prepared statistical plan. We have relied on the good offices of a
number of pathologists in scattered parts of the country, who
send samples when local circumstances permit. For practical
reasons it has been necessary to institute some selection. The
death rate is highest in the elderly and newborn. Our interest in

monitoring is largely in children whose growth rate is high but whose mortality is low. Thus we have accepted whatever samples have been sent us of infants over a month old and children but have instituted a rationing scheme for the newborn and adults.

The Glasgow group have drawn their material largely from a regional children's hospital, and from practically all autopsies a sample has been obtained. Where the Glasgow and the A.E.A. series overlap in 1959 and 1960, the results are closely comparable (60).

The bone chosen for analysis has been the femur. In young infants one femur does not provide a sufficient mass of material, and several long bones are often analyzed. In the very young there is no difference in concentration between bones. In children and adults one whole femur or longitudinal hemisection provides an excess of ash. Either a sample of the mixed ash is assayed, or, if only part of the bone is available, the sample is chosen to contain ivory and spongy bone; the former is preferred.

The results as reported have been summarized in Figure 39.

Adults.—From Figure 39 it will be noted that there has been a substantially constant level of strontium 90 in the adult's femur from 1956 to 1959. Differences between these years are not statistically significant. In 1960 the level rose to 0.3 $\mu\mu$c/g Ca. Thus, while the rate of fallout was constant and the concentration of strontium 90 in food was rising but slowly, the level of strontium 90 in the adults' femora was steady. Between May, 1958, and July, 1959, the rate of fallout was approximately three times the former rate, and dietary levels rose in 1959. The rise was reflected in bone in 1960.

The conditions in the normal adult are also reflected in the newborn infant, which has derived all its nutrients from maternal plasma. Owing to placental discrimination the specific activity per gram of calcium will be lower than in maternal plasma. Thus the observed values for bones of stillborn and newborn infants were 0.44 $\mu\mu$c/gm Ca (4 samples only) in 1956 and 0.6 $\mu\mu$c/gm Ca in 1957 and 1958, and in each year the level in maternal plasma must have been in the region of 1 $\mu\mu$c/gm Ca. Nevertheless, if

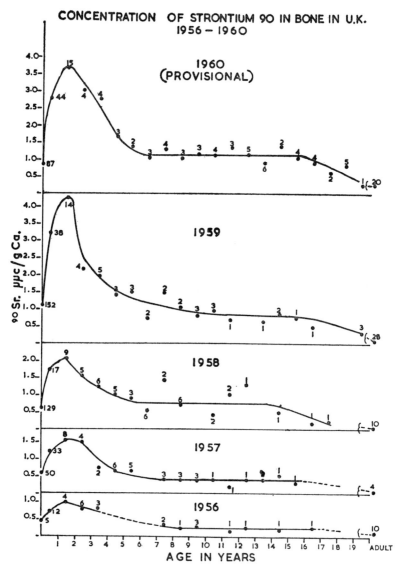

FIG. 39.—The mean specific activity of bone (femur) as μμc of strontium 90 per gram of calcium according to age in the years 1956–60. (Data
from United Kingdom.)

these mothers are representative of the adult population, adults' femora averaged only one-tenth of this concentration throughout the period. Our explanation of this was that only a fraction of the total femur can be exchanging mineral with plasma. It is extremely unlikely that all of this fraction is the conventional exchangeable mineral, which according to Bauer and others is only some 3–5 gm of the bone calcium in the whole body. Therefore, we postulate that the bone being replaced in turnover constitutes about one-tenth of the femur and that the same tenth keeps on turning over, leaving the remainder static.

In 1959 the concentration of strontium 90 in the newborn was about double that of the previous years. The Agricultural Research Council's figures for the national diet were some 50 per cent up on those of the preceding year. We could be confident that the concentration in the plasma of the average adult would have risen in 1959 by 50 to 100 per cent. Measurements in the plasma of an individual are not possible because of the extremely low concentration there. On the presumed levels the analyst would require something in excess of 20 liters of plasma, or 6 times as much as the average adult has in circulation at any one time. My colleagues (61) therefore analyzed in the winter of 1958–59 two pools of human plasma obtained but unsuitable for transfusion. The results were 1.1 and 1.4 $\mu\mu c/gm$ Ca. These are possibly underestimates, and higher levels would be expected in the spring and later.

Thus we would have predicted from our hypothesis that the concentration of strontium 90 in the adult's femur would rise later in 1959 or in 1960 from equilibrium of the 10 per cent or so pool of rapid turnover with plasma. The results for 1960 confirm a rise in that year. Naturally further years of observing levels in diet will be required to obtain a more definite picture. The values in diet had already fallen in 1960 and, if there were no further releases of fission products to the atmosphere from megaton devices, should have continued to fall slowly. A pool of rapid turnover would reflect this, but a larger pool of slow turnover could offset the loss.*

* Further weapon tests liberated fission products into the atmosphere in the autumn of 1961, so that no long period of steadily declining rates of deposition of strontium 90 will be available for consideration.

Children.—In contrast to adults, children showed (Fig. 40) a progressive rise in the concentration of strontium 90 in their femora with each year up to 1960. The youngest children have the highest levels in each year. In the full-grown adults all one has to consider is the replacement of existing bone with newly formed bone. In children there is growth in addition to remodeling. The annual growth in absolute terms and relative to the pre-existing skeletal mass can be derived from the standard values of Mitchell *et al.* given in Figure 37. Relative growth is maximal in the first years of life, falling off thereafter but making a slight comeback around puberty. In absolute values there are two modes, in early life and around puberty.

While we can be reasonably confident of this factor, we have hitherto not had any measure of the amount of remodeling each

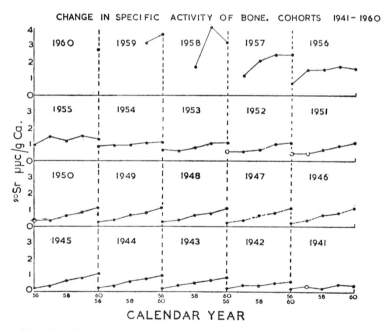

FIG. 40.—The mean specific activity of bone (femur) as μμc of strontium 90 per gram of calcium for the 20 cohorts born 1941 to 1960 in the calendar years 1956–60. (Data from United Kingdom.)

year of the existing bone. From general physiological principles one would expect it to be considerable, particularly in the early formative years. It was, therefore, surprising that Kulp and his colleagues (62) in their calculations relating to the uptake of strontium 90 by bone assumed a constant factor for turnover, namely the same value of about 3 per cent per annum that they had deduced from their data for adults. Having the advantage over Kulp of measures of strontium 90 relative to stable strontium as well as calcium, we have estimated the amount of annual replacement in preference to assuming it.

The observed values for stable strontium in the bones of infants and children are given in Figure 38. This shows an average value for the newborn of 200 μg/gm Ca, rising during the first year of life to about 260, after which it remains substantially constant till puberty. Thereafter the rise to the adult value of 320 must occur, though the observations in adolescence are scanty. The data are, however, adequate in the range of ages 1–10, for which we take the constant value of 260 μg/gm Ca.

The figures for strontium 90 in 1958 and 1959 are taken from the measurements of 1- to 10-year-old children in those years.

We thus have the specific activity, Sr^{90}/Sr, for children of each cohort born from 1949 to 1959. We have deduced from the available data the specific activity, Sr^{90}/Sr, of diet for each cohort in 1958 and 1959 (Table 6).

Consider the representative child of the 1957 cohort born at the midyear and aged 1 at the midpoint of 1958, when it has in its skeleton 100 gm. of calcium, 26.0 mg. of strontium and 200 $\mu\mu c$. of strontium 90. In the course of the next year, partly on the diet appropriate for 1958 of specific activity, 11.8 $\mu\mu c$/mg, and partly on that for 1959, 17 $\mu\mu c$/mg, it grows so that by mid-1959 the values for its skeleton are 147 gm. Ca, 38.2 mg. Sr, and 441 $\mu\mu c$. Sr^{90}. The increment of 12.2 mg. of strontium and 241 $\mu\mu c$. of strontium 90 indicates a specific activity of 20, about 50 per cent greater than the deduced mean specific activity of the diet. While this is not impossible due to the many uncertainties, the more probable explanation is that growth is accompanied by turnover of the

TABLE 6

ANNUAL RATE OF BONE TURNOVER CALCULATED FROM SPECIFIC ACTIVITIES*

COHORT	OBSERVED MEAN SPECIFIC ACTIVITY OF BONE				DEDUCED MEAN S.A. OF DIET (Sr⁹⁰μμc/mg Sr)		CALCULATED PERCENTAGE LIMITS OF PRE-EXISTING BONE REPLACED IN THE YEAR JULY 1958–JUNE 1959
	1959		1958				
	$Sr^{90}\mu\mu c/$ g Ca	$Sr^{90}\mu\mu c/$ mg Sr	$Sr^{90}\mu\mu c/$ g Ca	$Sr^{90}\mu\mu c/$ mg Sr	1958	1959	
1949....	0.85	3.4	0.70	2.7	7.7	11.3	0
1950....	0.9	3.5	0.75	2.9	7.9	11.5	0
1951....	1.0	3.8	0.75	3.0	8.2	12.0	0–8
1952....	1.1	4.1	0.8	3.1	8.5	12.3	3–13
1953....	1.2	4.6	0.95	3.6	8.9	12.9	2–12
1954....	1.4	5.4	1.1	4.3	9.2	13.3	4–14
1955....	1.8	6.8	1.4	5.4	9.7	13.7	9–28
1956....	2.2	8.3	1.85	7.1	10.0	14.3	0–35
1957....	3.0	12.3	2.0	8.1	11.8	17.0	14–91
1958....	4.3	16.5	0.62	3.1	?	?	—
1959....	1.13	5.65	—				

* Based upon table in F. J. Bryant and J. F. Loutit, *Human Bone Metabolism Deduced from Strontium Assays.* AERE-R 3718 (London, 1961).

existing bone as well as accretion. The amount of replacement of old bone by new bone with the same specific activity as the diet can be calculated. Two limits are derived, (*a*) the lower one for the whole diet at the deduced level for 1958, and (*b*) the upper one for the whole diet at the 1959 level. If *y* is the fraction of pre-existing bone not replaced in turnover:

μμc. Sr^{90} in mid-1959 = μμc. Sr^{90} accreted 1958–59
    $+ y$ (μμc. Sr^{90} mid-1958) $+ (1 - y)$ μμc. Sr^{90} replaced 1958–59.
Thus (*a*) $441 = 12.2 \times 11.8 + 200\,y + 26\,(1 - y) \times 11.8$
      ∴ $y = .09$ and $(1 - y) = .91$
   (*b*) $441 = 12.1 \times 17 + 200\,y + 26\,(1 - y) \times 17$
      ∴ $y = 0.86$ and $1 - y = 0.14$

Similar calculations were made for other cohorts and the results are given in last column of Table 6 and indicate a substantial turnover between the ages of 1 and 2, falling off to zero about the age of 7. The observations are not sufficiently numerous to allow calculations in the years of adolescence. One can say, however, that if turnover of pre-existing bone was considerable in adolescents one should have found a notable rise in concentration of bone in 1959 when the diet was contaminated to a considerably greater extent than formerly; no such rise was seen in the few specimens available.

At the other end of the range, if the proportion of pre-existing bone replaced is high in the second year of life, it is almost certainly higher in the first year. Because of the variations in methods of infant feeding, we did not feel justified in deriving representative diets for this age group. It is quite possible, however, as we pointed out, that there is complete replacement of pre-existing bone in this year which is the period of greatest proportional increase in skeletal mass. There would certainly need to be complete resorption of existing bone; what is uncertain is whether or not the existing bone salt is reutilized preferentially to mineral supplied from plasma.

The other phenomenon of importance in the formative years of life is the behavior of strontium relative to calcium. Has the child the same discriminatory powers as the adult? Kulp and his colleagues (62) in discussing the significance of their results obtained by survey of human bone assume that the discrimination shown by the adult applies also to the child. This over-all discrimination is assessed by Comar's observed ratio:

$$\frac{(\text{Sr/Ca in bone})}{(\text{Sr/Ca in diet})}.$$

A prerequisite for the right use of this ratio is that the bone being measured is in fact derived from the diet. The best situation is that utilized experimentally, feeding animals for a set period of time on diets of radioactive isotopes of strontium and calcium where the ratio of isotopes is known and then estimating the ratio of those isotopes in bone. The convention is also used in surveys. Thus adults are assumed to have been on the same diet for years, so that their bones will have come into equilibrium with it. If this assumption is correct, and it may not be, the national British diet, we have noted, is estimated to have a strontium:calcium ratio of 1.3 mg/gm Ca. The average of the ratio in adult bone is 0.32 mg/gm giving an observed ratio of ∼0.25, similar to that of experimental animals on labeled diets. If in fact this 1.3 mg/gm is an underestimate for diet, the true observed ratio will be lower.

When we turn to infants, since we believe their bone turnover is great and that, furthermore, most of their bone is newly accreted, we can derive observed ratios. At the age of both 1 and 2 the average value of bone is 260 µg/gm and the diets, according to my calculations from Widdowson, are 500 and 580 mg. Sr:0.9 gm. Ca, which give observed ratios of 0.5 and 0.4; that is, much higher than in the adult. Comar would predict, from his experimental evidence of facilitated intestinal uptake of strontium by amino acids and lactose, that this should happen with diets based on milk.

With children older than 2 years of age the observed ratio should not be derived directly from values of bone and diets. Rates of accretion and turnover have fallen, so that bone is a mélange of recently and remotely formed mineral. What we can say is that the ratio of strontium to calcium in bone stays constant up to the age of 10, while the ratio in diet is calculated to be rising. Thus during this period the observed ratio must be falling.

Some estimates can also be made from the survey of strontium 90. In Britain, unlike the U.S.A., infant feeding is not by standard formula. Breast feeding is universally recommended by pediatricians but practiced much less and for variable lengths of time by mothers. Both fresh cow's milk and dried milks are used for artificial feeding. Breast milk according to observations in the U.S.A. (Lough *et al.* [44]) has a strontium 90:calcium ratio of about 10 per cent of the lactating women's diet. In Britain in 1959, therefore, breast milk should have had a concentration of about 1 µµc/gm calcium. Fresh cow's milk averaged 7–15 µµc/gm calcium according to region, with a national mean of 10. Dried milk as purchased may have been somewhat lower due to earlier production. Such other infant foods as were measured were also lower. Thus 10 µµc.

of strontium 90 per gram of calcium is likely to have been a maximum figure for the diet of the representative infant. The analyses of bones of infants in the latter half of their first year of life gave averages of 4 $\mu\mu c$/gm calcium. Thus a minimum value for the observed ratio would be 0.4.

Since the over-all discrimination indicated by the observed ratio is a product normally of intestinal and renal discrimination, a raised observed ratio must mean decrease of intestinal discrimination or renal discrimination or both. The observations in newborn infants of Widdowson and that group previously referred to suggested fully active renal discrimination; therefore poor intestinal discrimination is the likely cause.

For children of the age of 1 and over, I have calculated elsewhere that the ratio of strontium 90 to calcium should not exceed that in the national British diet. Thus 1-year-olds with a strontium 90:calcium ratio in bone of 4 in 1959 and a ratio in diet of $\sim$10 also give an observed ratio of about 0.4. If this value were maintained in subsequent years, one would conclude that infants of the 1956 cohort would in 1958 have strontium 90:calcium ratios in their bones equal to or greater than infants of the 1958 cohort. In fact in each year of observation so far, the peak value has been recorded in the 1-year-olds. This would be expected in 1959 because of the pronounced increase in strontium 90 in fresh foods and the national diet in 1959 and late 1958, but it should not have been the case in 1957 and 1958 unless the observed ratio begins to fall after the second year of life.

To conclude I will attempt to summarize my present views about the growth and turnover of the skeleton with particular emphasis on strontium.

1. The newborn child is born with about 30 gm. of calcium in the body and a strontium concentration of 200 μg/gm Ca. It has an urgent need for phosphate for its soft tissue and, if the diet is marginally adequate in phosphate, as in breast milk, calcium and strontium phosphates are withdrawn from the skeleton. Calcium is preserved by the body, but a negative balance of strontium may result.

2. The infant's kidneys are mature enough to discriminate between calcium and strontium, but the intestinal mucosa may be less forward. Thus the total discrimination by the infant's metabolic processes favoring retention of calcium and discharge of strontium may be less than in later life.

3. During growth in infancy there is a remarkably fast accretion of mineral into the skeleton—a threefold increase in the first year of life. Necessarily there is complete remodeling of the bones. Exactly how much of the original mineral is reutilized is uncertain, but most of the mineral at the end of the first year must have been derived from dietary sources. The concentration of strontium (and strontium 90) in terms of calcium will be about one half that in the diet: In the United Kingdom it is now about 260 μg (and 3–4 $\mu\mu c$ Sr^{90}) per gram of calcium for the representative 1-year-old.

3. With increasing years the rate of accretion of new bone mineral and of turnover of existing mineral falls off. At the same time the faculty of discrimination between strontium and calcium increases. Thus by about the age of 7, the skeletal mass has increased rather less than threefold since the age of 1, but the strontium concentration remains about the same at 260 $\mu g/gm$ Ca, and the strontium 90 concentration is less than in infancy.

4. From this time onward the rate of accretion of new bone mineral rises again, but remodeling seems to be minimal. Thus growth round the age of puberty is largely a plastering on of new salt. Probably about this time the increasing concentration of stable strontium (but not strontium 90) in the diet leads to an increase in stable strontium concentration in the skeleton toward the adult value (for the U.K.) of 320 $\mu g/gm$ Ca.

5. About puberty also, probably associated with the changes in activities of endocrine glands, the relative distribution of absorbed calcium and strontium between bone and excreta alters markedly so that these absorbed minerals are shunted more to excreta and less to bone.

The concentration of strontium 90 in bone up till now is therefore related to the proportion of the total life span which has been spent in contaminated surroundings with contaminated food; that is, there has been a progressive fall with age.

6. On reaching adult life true accretion of bone mineral ceases, but a certain amount of maintenance or replacement continues. In the healthy subject absorption of calcium and strontium just balances excretion: normally in the elderly, however, and at all ages in demineralizing diseases there may be a net loss of minerals.

From observations with radioactive isotopes of calcium and strontium, an understanding of the dynamics of the mineral metabolism is being attained, though as yet it is far from complete. The observations may be from planned experiments in the laboratory or from survey data acquired from the monitoring of strontium 90, the first universal tracer study with man-made radioactive material.

The planned experiments would suggest that the gross apposition of new mineral in the skeleton amounts to about one-half a gram of calcium and several hundreds of micrograms of strontium a day. This is conceived as drawn from a soft tissue plus fluid pool which is topped up by absorption from the gut and drained by excretion to urine and feces.

Rapid ion exchange between the fluid pool and the surface of accessible bone crystals occurs. In these accessible areas the apposition of new bone by crystallization is probably occurring. This provides a further surface for exchange in virtue of the small size of recently formed crystals; it probably also buries some surfaces formerly available. The recently formed crystals are, however, imperfect. The imperfections have to be made good and this is done by exchange between atoms on the surface with others beneath—intracrystalline exchange. Maturation of the newly formed bone occurs, probably associated with recrystallization; until the bone is fully mature there is always opportunity for atoms of calcium and strontium originally incorporated in the primary crystals to escape and be replaced. It is suggested that the return of this evanescent scaffolding-type of mineral accounts in part for the apparently changing rate of uptake with time of a single dose of a radioactive marker. An alternate explanation which has been propounded is that there is a poorly accessible space in bone into which ions from the fluid pool can diffuse in and out slowly.[2] The gross rate of uptake therefore probably overestimates true bone-formation rate.

Furthermore from the evidence of survey data we conclude that some bone units have a relatively short life span, some longer, and some a very long span before being replaced. The short-lived bone units may be replaced several times within the year and be in equilibrium with the fluid pool as far as strontium 90 is concerned, whereas many of the long-lived units have not yet taken up any strontium 90. Cancellous bone, particularly of the spine, seems to be composed of shorter-lived units, whereas ivory bone, like the shaft of the femur and skullcap, is mainly of long-lived units. This would be in accord with classical observations that when there is a drain on the body's mineral stores (e.g., during lactation) it is cancellous bones which demineralize first.

---

[2] If this were the case the apparent size of the fluid pool would expand until the second diffusion space was in equilibrium. From a current experiment in which markers are given daily with food for a month, we have detected little sign of this expanding exchange space.

References

1. PECHER, C. Univ. California Publ. Pharmacol. 2 (No. 11): 117. 1942.
2. HAMILTON, J. G. Radiology, 49: 325. 1947.
3. BRUES, A. M. J. Clin. Invest., 28: 1286. 1949.
4. FINKEL, M. P.; BISKIS, B. O.; and SCRIBNER, G. M. *In:* Progress in Nuclear Energy VI Biological Sciences 2, ed. J. C. BUGHER, J. COURSAGET, and J. F. LOUTIT, p. 199. Pergamon Press, London. 1959.
5. MARINELLI, L. D. Amer. J. Roentgenol., 80: 729. 1958.
6. HASTERLIK, R. F. Proc. Int. Conf. Peaceful Uses of Atomic Energy. United Nations, New York, 11: 149. 1956.
7. MARTLAND, H. S. Amer. J. Cancer, 15: 2435. 1931.
8. AUB, J. C.; EVANS, R. D.; HEMPELMANN, L. H.; and MARTLAND, H. S. Medicine, 31: 221. 1952.
9. HARRISON, G. E.; RAYMOND, W. H. A.; and TRETHEWAY, H. C. Clin. Sci., 14: 681. 1955.
10. HARRISON, G. E., and RAYMOND, W. H. A. J. Nuc. Energy, 1: 290. 1955.
11. HARRISON, G. E. Nature (Lond.), 182: 792. 1958.
12. COMAR, C. L.; WASSERMAN, R. H.; ULLBERG, S.; and ANDREWS, G. A. Proc. Soc. Exp. Biol. (N.Y.), 95: 386. 1957.
13. LASZLO, D., and SPENCER, H. *In:* Progress in Nuclear Energy VII Medical Sciences 2, ed. J. C. BUGHER, J. COURSAGET, and J. F. LOUTIT, p. 151. Pergamon Press, London. 1959.
14. RYGH, O. Bull Soc. Chim. Biol., 31: 1052. 1949.
15. INTERNATIONAL COMMISSION ON RADIOLOGICAL PROTECTION. Report of Sub-committee II. Brit. J. Radiol., Supp. 6, 23. 1955.
16. NAORA, H.; NAORA, H.; MIRSKY, A. E.; and ALLFREY, V. G. J. Gen. Physiol., 44: 713. 1961.
17. BAUER, G. C. H.; CARLSSON, A.; and LINDQUIST, B. Acta med. scand., 158: 143. 1957.
18. NEUMAN, W. F., and NEUMAN, M. W. The Chemical Dynamics of Bone Mineral. Univ. Chicago Press. 1958.
19. AMPRINO, R., and ENGSTRÖM, A. Acta anat., 15: 1. 1952.
20. BAUER, G. C. H.; CARLSSON, A.; and LINDQUIST, B. *In:* Mineral Metabolism, ed. C. L. COMAR and F. BRONNER. Vol. 1, Part B, p. 609. Academic Press, New York. 1961.
21. BAUER, G. C. H., and RAY, R. D. J. Bone & Joint Surg. 40: 171. 1958.
22. MINISTRY OF AGRICULTURE, FISHERIES AND FOOD. Domestic Food Consumption and Expenditure 1957. H.M.S.O., London. 1959.

23. McCance, R. A., and Widdowson, E. M. M.R.C. Special Report Series, No. 235. H.M.S.O., London. 1942.
24. Chen, P. S., and Neuman, W. F. Amer. J. Physiol., 180: 623, 632. 1955.
25. Carter, C. W.; Coxon, R. V.; Parsons, D. S.; and Thompson, R.H.S. Biochemistry in Relation to Medicine, 3d ed., p. 246. Longmans Green, London. 1959.
26. Irving, J. T. Calcium Metabolism. Methuen, London. 1957.
27. Duckworth, J., and Hill, R. Nutr. Abstr. & Rev., 23: 1. 1953.
28. Nordin, B. E. C. Lancet, 1: 1011. 1961.
29. Harrison, M.; Fraser, R.; and Mullan, B. Lancet, 1: 1015. 1961.
30. Agricultural Research Council Radiobiological Laboratory. Report No. 1. H.M.S.O., London. 1959.
31. Harrison, G. E. Unpublished data.
32. Loutit, J. F. Irish J. Med. Sci., No. 427, 6th series, 283. 1961.
33. Comar, C. L.; Russell, R. S.; and Wasserman, R. H. Science, 126: 485. 1957.
34. Russell, R. S., and Squire, H. J. Exp. Bot., 9: 262. 1958.
35. Cramer, C. F., and Copp, D. H. Proc. Soc. Exp. Biol. (N.Y.), 102: 514. 1959
36. Schachter, D.; Dowdle, E. B.; and Schenker, H. Amer. J. Physiol. 198: 263. 1960.
37. Wasserman, R. H. Proc. Soc. Exp. Biol. (N.Y.), 104: 92. 1960.
38. Dumont, P. A.; Curran, P. F.; and Solomon, A. K. J. Gen. Physiol., 43: 1119. 1960.
39. Bishop, M.; Harrison, G. E.; Raymond, W. H. A.; Sutton, A. and Rundo, J. Internat. J. Rad. Biol. 2: 125. 1960.
40. Steggerda, F. R., and Mitchell, H. H. J. Nutrit., 31: 432. 1946.
41. Spencer, H.; Li, M.; Samachson, J.; and Laszlo, D. Metabolism, 9: 916. 1960.
42. Barnes, D. W. H., Bishop, M., Harrison, G. E.; and Sutton, A. Internat. J. Rad. Biol., 3: 637. 1961.
43. Mitchell, H. H., and Hamilton, T. S. J. Biol. Chem., 178: 345. 1949.
44. Lough, S. Allan; Hamada, G. H.; and Comar, C. L. Proc. Soc. Exp. Biol. (N.Y.), 104: 194. 1960.
45. Bryant, F. J., and Loutit, J. F. A.E.R.E. R–3718. H.M.S.O., London. 1961.
46. Stewart, C. G.; Vogt, E.; Hitchman, A. J. W.; and Jupe, N. *In:* Progress in Nuclear Energy, VII Medical Sciences, 2, ed. J. C. Bugher, J. Coursaget, and J. F. Loutit, p. 39. Pergamon Press. London. 1959.

47. RUNDO, J., and WILLIAMS, K. Brit. J. Radiol. (in press).
48. BLUHM, M.; MACGREGOR, J.; and NORDIN, B. E. C. Radioaktiv Isotope in Klinik und Forschung. **IV**: 29. 1960.
49. HEANEY, R. P., and WHEDON, G. D. J. Clin. Endocrinol., **18**: 1246. 1958.
50. LACROIX, P. Experientia, **8**: 426. 1952.
51. JOWSEY, J.; OWEN, M.; and VAUGHAN, J. Brit. J. Exp. Path., **34**: 661. 1953.
52. MARSHALL, J. H. *In:* Bone as a Tissue, ed. K. RODAHL, J. T. NICHOLSON, and E. M. BROWN, p. 144. McGraw-Hill Book Co., New York. 1960.
53. MITCHELL, H. H.; STEGGERDA, F. R.; and BEAN, H. W. J. Biol. Chem., **158**: 625. 1945.
54. WIDDOWSON, E. M. Medical Research Council Special Report Series, No. 257. H.M.S.O., London. 1947.
55. WIDDOWSON, E. M.; SLATER, J. E.; HARRISON, G. E.; and SUTTON, A. Lancet, **2**: 941. 1960.
56. BEDFORD, JOAN; HARRISON, G. E.; RAYMOND, W. H. A.; and SUTTON, A. Brit. Med. J. **1**: 589. 1960.
57. AGRICULTURAL RESEARCH COUNCIL RADIOBIOLOGICAL LABORATORY. A.R.C.R.L. 1,2,3,4, and 5. H.M.S.O., London. 1959, 1960, 1960, 1961, 1961.
58. BRYANT, F. J.; CHAMBERLAIN, A. C.; SPICER, G. S.; and WEBB, M. S. W. Brit. Med. J., **1**: 1371. 1958.
59. LOUTIT, J. F.; MARLEY, W. G.; MAYNEORD, W. V.; and RUSSELL, R. S. Appendix F. *In:* Hazards to Man of Nuclear and Allied Radiations. Cmnd. 1225. H.M.S.O., London. 1960.
60. BRYANT, F. J.; HENDERSON, E. H.; LEA, I.; LLOYD, G. D., and WEBB, M. S. W. Medical Research Council Monitoring Report Series No. 1 and No. 2. H.M.S.O., London. 1961.
61. HARRISON, G. E.; SUTTON, A.; and MAYCOCK, W. D'A. Nature (Lond.), **189**: 324. 1961.
62. KULP, J. L.; SCHULERT, A. R.; and HODGES, E. J. Science, **132**: 448. 1960.

SUBJECT INDEX

α-rays; *see* Radiation
Abortion, threatened, 65
Absorption by gut, 102–5, 108, 113, 115, 126, 130, 138, 141
Absorptive discrimination, 111, 139, 140
Activation analysis, 90
Active transport, 108
Adaptation, 103–7
Adrenals, 45, 105
Adults
    Sr^{90} contamination in, 131, 133
    stable strontium in, 115, 130, 135, 140
Aging
    accelerated, 35–36
    development of, 36, 39
    experimental, 27–44
    natural, 17–22
    premature, 28, 36
    and radiation, 22–27
Amniotic fluid, 125
Anemia, 24, 67, 89
Ankylosing spondylitis, 76, 78–79
Apatite, 93, 95
Artificial feeding, 125, 138
Atom bomb, 41, 74–79, 127
Atrophy, 14
    of thymus, 55
Availability, 108, 113, 130

β-rays; *see* Radiation
Background; *see* Radiation
Bacteria, 15, 21, 46
Bacteriology, 17
Balance studies, 101–7, 110, 113, 124–26, 139
Barium, 89, 110
Bicarbonate, 92, 95
"Biochemical lesion," 7
Biochemistry, 2
Biological assay, 58
Biological targets, 3–5
Blood
    -bone relations, 115
    plasma (serum), 92, 98–99, 104–5, 109, 111–21, 131, 133, 137

Bone
    apposition (accretion), 93, 96–97, 99, 110, 102, 115–18, 120, 122, 136, 138, 140–41
    cancellous (trabecular), 93, 96–97, 104, 121, 131, 142
    erosion (resorption), 93, 96–97, 137
    exchangeable, 94–97, 99, 100, 117, 120, 133
    femur, 131–35, 142
    fracture, 89
    ivory, 93, 96–97, 121, 131, 142
    long, 93
    maturation, 97, 120, 141
    necrosis, 24, 89
    non-exchangeable, 94, 100
    radioactivity in, 24, 88 *et seq.*
    sarcoma, 24, 89
    see also Bone marrow
Bone marrow, 4, 7, 14, 15, 24, 47–49, 51, 77, 89
    factor, 60
    reseeding, 61
    shielding, 60, 62
Break; *see* Chromosomes
Breast feeding, 123, 125, 138
Breast tissue; *see* Mammary glands
Bronchi; *see* Lung

Calcium, 89, 90, 91–105, 106–15, 117, 119, 120, 122, 123–24, 126–29, 131–32, 135, 137
Calculation of
    availability of strontium, 107
    bone-formation rate, 99–101
    bone turnover, 135–36
    exchange space 99–101
    exogenous-endogenous differences, 110
    strontium in children's diet, 129–30
Cancer, 5–8, 10, 15, 18, 21–22, 34, 40–41, 44–82, 89, 113
    see also under specific organs
Carcinogenic agents, 45, 60, 68, 73
Carriers, 59

147

NAME INDEX